The Next Generation: Third Wave Feminist Psychotherapy

The Next Generation: Third Wave Feminist Psychotherapy has been co-published simultaneously as *Women & Therapy*, Volume 23, Number 2 2001.

The *Women & Therapy* Monographic "Separates"

Below is a list of "separates," which in serials librarianship means a special issue simultaneously published as a special journal issue or double-issue *and* as a "separate" hardbound monograph. (This is a format which we also call a "DocuSerial.")

"Separates" are published because specialized libraries or professionals may wish to purchase a specific thematic issue by itself in a format which can be separately cataloged and shelved, as opposed to purchasing the journal on an on-going basis. Faculty members may also more easily consider a "separate" for classroom adoption.

"Separates" are carefully classified separately with the major book jobbers so that the journal tie-in can be noted on new book order slips to avoid duplicate purchasing.

You may wish to visit Haworth's website at . . .

http://www.HaworthPress.com

. . . to search our online catalog for complete tables of contents of these separates and related publications.

You may also call 1-800-HAWORTH (outside US/Canada: 607-722-5857), or Fax 1-800-895-0582 (outside US/Canada: 607-771-0012), or e-mail at:

getinfo@haworthpressinc.com

The Next Generation: Third Wave Feminist Psychotherapy, edited by Ellyn Kaschak, PhD (Vol. 23, No. 2, 2001). *Discusses the issues young feminists face, focusing on the implications for psychotherapists of the false sense that feminism is no longer necessary.*

Minding the Body: Psychotherapy in Cases of Chronic and Life-Threatening Illness, edited by Ellyn Kaschac, PhD (Vol. 23, No. 1, 2001). *Being diagnosed with cancer, lupus, or fibromyalgia is a traumatic event. All too often, women are told their disease is 'all in their heads' and therefore both 'unreal and insignificant' by a medical profession that dismisses emotions and scorns mental illness. Combining personal narratives and theoretical views of illness, Minding the Body offers an alternative approach to the mind-body connection. This book shows the reader how to deal with the painful and difficult emotions that exacerbate illness, while learning the emotional and spiritual lessons illness can teach.*

For Love or Money: The Fee in Feminist Therapy, edited by Marcia Hill, EdD, and Ellyn Kaschak, PhD (Vol. 22, No. 3, 1999). *"Recommended reading for both new and seasoned professionals. . . . An exciting and timely book about 'the last taboo'. . . . " (Carolyn C. Larsen, PhD, Senior Counsellor Emeritus, University of Calgary; Partner, Alberta Psychological Resources Ltd., Calgary, and Co-editor, Ethical Decision Making in Therapy: Feminist Perspectives)*

Beyond the Rule Book: Moral Issues and Dilemmas in the Practice of Psychotherapy, edited by Ellyn Kaschak, PhD, and Marcia Hill, EdD (Vol. 22, No. 2, 1999). *"The authors in this important and timely book tackle the difficult task of working through . . . conflicts, sharing their moral struggles and real life solutions in working with diverse populations and in a variety of clinical settings. . . . Will provide psychotherapists with a thought-provoking source for the stimulating and essential discussion of our own and our profession's moral bases." (Carolyn C. Larsen, PhD, Senior Counsellor Emeritus, University of Calgary, Partner in private practice, Alberta Psychological Resources Ltd., Calgary, and Co-editor, Ethical Decision Making in Therapy: Feminist Perspectives)*

Assault on the Soul: Women in the Former Yugoslavia, edited by Sara Sharratt, PhD, and Ellyn Kaschak, PhD (Vol. 22, No. 1, 1999). *Explores the applications and intersections of feminist therapy, activism and jurisprudence with women and children in the former Yugoslavia.*

Learning from Our Mistakes: Difficulties and Failures in Feminist Therapy, edited by Marcia Hill, EdD, and Esther D. Rothblum, PhD (Vol. 21, No. 3, 1998). *"A courageous and fundamental step in evolving a well-grounded body of theory and of investigating the assumptions that unexamined, lead us to error." (Teresa Bernardez, MD, Training and Supervising Analyst, The Michigan Psychoanalytic Council)*

Feminist Therapy as a Political Act, edited by Marcia Hill, EdD (Vol. 21, No. 2, 1998). *"A real contribution to the field. . . . A valuable tool for feminist therapists and those who want to learn about feminist therapy." (Florence L. Denmark, PhD, Robert S. Pace Distinguished Professor of Psychology and Chair, Psychology Department, Pace University, New York, New York)*

Breaking the Rules: Women in Prison and Feminist Therapy, edited by Judy Harden, PhD, and Marcia Hill, EdD (Vol. 20, No. 4 & Vol. 21, No. 1, 1998). *"Fills a long-recognized gap in the psychology of women curricula, demonstrating that feminist theory can be made relevant to the practice of feminism, even in prison." (Suzanne J. Kessler, PhD, Professor of Psychology and Women's Studies, State University of New York at Purchase)*

Children's Rights, Therapists' Responsibilities: Feminist Commentaries, edited by Gail Anderson, MA, and Marcia Hill, EdD (Vol. 20, No. 2, 1997). *"Addresses specific practice dimensions that will help therapists organize and resolve conflicts about working with children, adolescents, and their families in therapy." (Feminist Bookstore News)*

More than a Mirror: How Clients Influence Therapists' Lives, edited by Marcia Hill, EdD (Vol. 20, No. 1, 1997). *"Courageous, insightful, and deeply moving. These pages reveal the scrupulous self-examination and self-reflection of conscientious therapists at their best. AN IMPORTANT CONTRIBUTION TO FEMINIST THERAPY LITERATURE AND A BOOK WORTH READING BY THERAPISTS AND CLIENTS ALIKE." (Rachel Josefowitz Siegal, MSW, retired feminist therapy practitioner; Co-Editor, Women Changing Therapy; Jewish Women in Therapy; and Celebrating the Lives of Jewish Women: Patterns in a Feminist Sampler)*

Sexualities, edited by Marny Hall, PhD, LCSW (Vol. 19, No. 4, 1997). *"Explores the diverse and multifaceted nature of female sexuality, covering topics including sadomasochism in the therapy room, sexual exploitation in cults, and genderbending in cyberspace." (Feminist Bookstore News)*

Couples Therapy: Feminist Perspectives, edited by Marcia Hill, EdD, and Esther D. Rothblum, PhD (Vol. 19, No. 3, 1996). *Addresses some of the inadequacies, omissions, and assumptions in traditional couples' therapy to help you face the issues of race, ethnicity, and sexual orientation in helping couples today.*

A Feminist Clinician's Guide to the Memory Debate, edited by Susan Contratto, PhD, and M. Janice Gutfreund, PhD (Vol. 19, No. 1, 1996). *"Unites diverse scholars, clinicians, and activists in an insightful and useful examination of the issues related to recovered memories." (Feminist Bookstore News)*

Classism and Feminist Therapy: Counting Costs, edited by Marcia Hill, EdD, and Esther D. Rothblum, PhD (Vol. 18, No. 3/4, 1996). *"EDUCATES, CHALLENGES, AND QUESTIONS THE INFLUENCE OF CLASSISM ON THE CLINICAL PRACTICE OF PSYCHOTHERAPY WITH WOMEN." (Kathleen P. Gates, MA, Certified Professional Counselor, Center for Psychological Health, Superior, Wisconsin)*

Lesbian Therapists and Their Therapy: From Both Sides of the Couch, edited by Nancy D. Davis, MD, Ellen Cole, PhD, and Esther D. Rothblum, PhD (Vol. 18, No. 2, 1996). *"Highlights the power and boundary issues of psychotherapy from perspectives that many readers may have neither considered nor experienced in their own professional lives." (Psychiatric Services)*

Feminist Foremothers in Women's Studies, Psychology, and Mental Health, edited by Phyllis Chesler, PhD, Esther D. Rothblum, PhD, and Ellen Cole, PhD (Vol. 17, No. 1/2/3/4, 1995). *"A must for feminist scholars and teachers . . . These women's personal experiences are poignant and powerful." (Women's Studies International Forum)*

Women's Spirituality, Women's Lives, edited by Judith Ochshorn, PhD, and Ellen Cole, PhD (Vol. 16, No. 2/3, 1995). *"A delightful and complex book on spirituality and sacredness in women's lives." (Joan Clingan, MA, Spiritual Psychology, Graduate Advisor, Prescott College Master of Arts Program)*

Psychopharmacology from a Feminist Perspective, edited by Jean A. Hamilton, MD, Margaret Jensvold, MD, Esther D. Rothblum, PhD, and Ellen Cole, PhD (Vol. 16, No. 1, 1995). *"Challenges readers to increase their sensitivity and awareness of the role of sex and gender in re-*

sponse to and acceptance of pharmacologic therapy." (American Journal of Pharmaceutical Education)

Wilderness Therapy for Women: The Power of Adventure, edited by Ellen Cole, PhD, Esther D. Rothblum, PhD, and Eve Erdman, MEd, MLS (Vol. 15, No. 3/4, 1994). *"There's an undeniable excitement in these pages about the thrilling satisfaction of meeting challenges in the physical world, the world outside our cities that is unfamiliar, uneasy territory for many women. If you're interested at all in the subject, this book is well worth your time."* (Psychology of Women Quarterly)

Bringing Ethics Alive: Feminist Ethics in Psychotherapy Practice, edited by Nanette K. Gartrell, MD (Vol. 15, No. 1, 1994). *"Examines the theoretical and practical issues of ethics in feminist therapies. From the responsibilities of training programs to include social issues ranging from racism to sexism to practice ethics, this outlines real questions and concerns."* (Midwest Book Review)

Women with Disabilities: Found Voices, edited by Mary Willmuth, PhD, and Lillian Holcomb, PhD (Vol. 14, No. 3/4, 1994). *"These powerful chapters often jolt the anti-disability consciousness and force readers to contend with the ways in which disability has been constructed, disguised, and rendered disgusting by much of society."* (Academic Library Book Review)

Faces of Women and Aging, edited by Nancy D. Davis, MD, Ellen Cole, PhD, and Esther D. Rothblum, PhD (Vol. 14, No. 1/2, 1993). *"This uplifting, helpful book is of great value not only for aging women, but also for women of all ages who are interested in taking active control of their own lives."* (New Mature Woman)

Refugee Women and Their Mental Health: Shattered Societies, Shattered Lives, edited by Ellen Cole, PhD, Oliva M. Espin, PhD, and Esther D. Rothblum, PhD (Vol. 13, No. 1/2/3, 1992). *"The ideas presented are rich and the perspectives varied, and the book is an important contribution to understanding refugee women in a global context."* (Comtemporary Psychology)

Women, Girls and Psychotherapy: Reframing Resistance, edited by Carol Gilligan, PhD, Annie Rogers, PhD, and Deborah Tolman, EdD (Vol. 11, No. 3/4, 1991). *"Of use to educators, psycho-therapists, and parents-in short, to any person who is directly involved with girls at adolescence."* (Harvard Educational Review)

Professional Training for Feminist Therapists: Personal Memoirs, edited by Esther D. Rothblum, PhD, and Ellen Cole, PhD (Vol. 11, No. 1, 1991). *"Exciting, interesting, and filled with the angst and the energies that directed these women to develop an entirely different approach to counseling."* (Science Books & Films)

Jewish Women in Therapy: Seen But Not Heard, edited by Rachel Josefowitz Siegel, MSW, and Ellen Cole, PhD (Vol. 10, No. 4, 1991). *"A varied collection of prose and poetry, first-person stories, and accessible theoretical pieces that can help Jews and non-Jews, women and men, therapists and patients, and general readers to grapple with questions of Jewish women's identities and diversity."* (Canadian Psychology)

Women's Mental Health in Africa, edited by Esther D. Rothblum, PhD, and Ellen Cole, PhD (Vol. 10, No. 3, 1990). *"A valuable contribution and will be of particular interest to scholars in women's studies, mental health, and cross-cultural psychology."* (Contemporary Psychology)

Motherhood: A Feminist Perspective, edited by Jane Price Knowles, MD, and Ellen Cole, PhD (Vol. 10, No. 1/2, 1990). *"Provides some enlightening perspectives. . . . It is worth the time of both male and female readers."* (Comtemporary Psychology)

Diversity and Complexity in Feminist Therapy, edited by Laura Brown, PhD, ABPP, and Maria P. P. Root, PhD (Vol. 9, No. 1/2, 1990). *"A most convincing discussion and illustration of the importance of adopting a multicultural perspective for theory building in feminist therapy. . . . THIS BOOK IS A MUST FOR THERAPISTS and should be included on psychology of women syllabi."* (Association for Women in Psychology Newsletter)

Fat Oppression and Psychotherapy, edited by Laura S. Brown, PhD, and Esther D. Rothblum, PhD (Vol. 8, No. 3, 1990). *"Challenges many traditional beliefs about being fat . . . A refreshing new* *perspective for approaching and thinking about issues related to weight." (Association for Women in Psychology Newsletter)*

Lesbianism: Affirming Nontraditional Roles, edited by Esther D. Rothblum, PhD, and Ellen Cole, PhD (Vol. 8, No. 1/2, 1989). *"Touches on many of the most significant issues brought before therapists today." (Newsletter of the Association of Gay & Lesbian Psychiatrists)*

Women and Sex Therapy: Closing the Circle of Sexual Knowledge, edited by Ellen Cole, PhD, and Esther D. Rothblum, PhD (Vol. 7, No. 2/3, 1989). *"ADDS IMMEASUREABLY TO THE FEMINIST THERAPY LITERATURE THAT DISPELS MALE PARADIGMS OF PATHOLOGY WITH REGARD TO WOMEN." (Journal of Sex Education & Therapy)*

The Politics of Race and Gender in Therapy, edited by Lenora Fulani, PhD (Vol. 6, No. 4, 1988). *Women of color examine newer therapies that encourage them to develop their historical identity.*

Treating Women's Fear of Failure, edited by Esther D. Rothblum, PhD, and Ellen Cole, PhD (Vol. 6, No. 3, 1988). *"SHOULD BE RECOMMENDED READING FOR ALL MENTAL HEALTH PROFESSIONALS, SOCIAL WORKERS, EDUCATORS, AND VOCATIONAL COUNSELORS WHO WORK WITH WOMEN." (The Journal of Clinical Psychiatry)*

Women, Power, and Therapy: Issues for Women, edited by Marjorie Braude, MD (Vol. 6, No. 1/2, 1987). *"RAISE[S] THERAPISTS' CONSCIOUSNESS ABOUT THE IMPORTANCE OF CONSIDERING GENDER-BASED POWER IN THERAPY. . . welcome contribution." (Australian Journal of Psychology)*

Dynamics of Feminist Therapy, edited by Doris Howard (Vol. 5, No. 2/3, 1987). *"A comprehensive treatment of an important and vexing subject." (Australian Journal of Sex, Marriage and Family)*

A Woman's Recovery from the Trauma of War: Twelve Responses from Feminist Therapists and Activists, edited by Esther D. Rothblum, PhD, and Ellen Cole, PhD (Vol. 5, No. 1, 1986). *"A MILESTONE. In it, twelve women pay very close attention to a woman who has been deeply wounded by war." (The World)*

Women and Mental Health: New Directions for Change, edited by Carol T. Mowbray, PhD, Susan Lanir, MA, and Marilyn Hulce, MSW, ACSW (Vol. 3, No. 3/4, 1985). *"The overview of sex differences in disorders is clear and sensitive, as is the review of sexual exploitation of clients by therapists. . . . MANDATORY READING FOR ALL THERAPISTS WHO WORK WITH WOMEN." (British Journal of Medical Psychology and The British Psychological Society)*

Women Changing Therapy: New Assessments, Values, and Strategies in Feminist Therapy, edited by Joan Hamerman Robbins and Rachel Josefowitz Siegel, MSW (Vol. 2, No. 2/3, 1983). *"An excellent collection to use in teaching therapists that reflection and resolution in treatment do not simply lead tp adaptation, but to an active inner process of judging." (News for Women in Psychiatry)*

Current Feminist Issues in Psychotherapy, edited by The New England Association for Women in Psychology (Vol. 1, No. 3, 1983). *Addresses depression, displaced homemakers, sibling incest, and body image from a feminist perspective.*

The Next Generation: Third Wave Feminist Psychotherapy

Ellyn Kaschak, PhD
Editor

The Next Generation: Third Wave Feminist Psychotherapy has been co-published simultaneously as *Women & Therapy*, Volume 23, Number 2 2001.

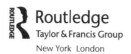

Routledge
Taylor & Francis Group
New York London

The Next Generation: Third Wave Feminist Psychotherapy has been co-published simultaneously as *Women & Therapy*™, Volume 23, Number 2 2001.

First published 2001 by The Haworth Press,Inc.

Published 2020 by Routledge
52 Vanderbilt Avenue, New York, NY 10017
2 Park Square, Milton Park, Abingdon, Oxon OX14 4RN

Routledge is an imprint of the Taylor & Francis Group, an informa business

Cover design by Thomas J. Mayshock Jr.

Library of Congress Cataloging-in-Publication Data

The next generation : third wave feminist psychotherapy/Ellyn Kaschak, editor.
 p. cm.
"... co-published simultaneously as Women & therapy, volume 23, number 2 2001."
Includes bibliographical references and index.
ISBN 0-7890-1409-2 (alk. paper) -- ISBN 0-7890-1410-6 (alk. paper)
1. Feminist therapy. 2. Psychotherapy. I. Kaschak, Ellyn, 1943-

RC489.F45 N495 20001
616.89´14´082--dc21

2001024982

ISBN 13: 978-0-7890-1410-8 (pbk)

Indexing, Abstracting & Website/Internet Coverage

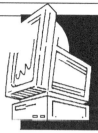

This section provides you with a list of major indexing & abstracting services. That is to say, each service began covering this periodical during the year noted in the right column. Most Websites which are listed below have indicated that they will either post, disseminate, compile, archive, cite or alert their own Website users with research-based content from this work. (This list is as current as the copyright date of this publication.)

(continued)

(continued)

Special Bibliographic Notes related to special journal issues (separates) and indexing/abstracting:

- indexing/abstracting services in this list will also cover material in any "separate" that is co-published simultaneously with Haworth's special thematic journal issue or DocuSerial. Indexing/abstracting usually covers material at the article/chapter level.
- monographic co-editions are intended for either non-subscribers or libraries which intend to purchase a second copy for their circulating collections.
- monographic co-editions are reported to all jobbers/wholesalers/approval plans. The source journal is listed as the "series" to assist the prevention of duplicate purchasing in the same manner utilized for books-in-series.
- to facilitate user/access services all indexing/abstracting services are encouraged to utilize the co-indexing entry note indicated at the bottom of the first page of each article/chapter/contribution.
- this is intended to assist a library user of any reference tool (whether print, electronic, online, or CD-ROM) to locate the monographic version if the library has purchased this version but not a subscription to the source journal.
- individual articles/chapters in any Haworth publication are also available through the Haworth Document Delivery Service (HDDS).

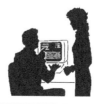

ABOUT THE EDITOR

Ellyn Kaschak, PhD, is Professor of Psychology at San Jose State University in San Jose, California. She is author of *Engendered Lives: A New Psychology of Women's Experience*, as well as numerous articles and chapters on feminist psychology and psychotherapy. Dr. Kaschak is editor of *Minding the Body: Psychotherapy in Cases of Chronic and Life-Threatening Illness* and co-editor of *Assault on the Soul: Women in the Former Yugoslavia*; *Beyond the Rule Book: Moral Issues and Dilemmas in the Practice of Psychotherapy*, and *For Love or Money: The Fee in Feminist Therapy*. She has had thirty years of experience practicing psychotherapy, is past Chair of the Feminist Therapy Institute and of the APA Committee on Women and is Fellow of Division 35, the Psychology of Women, Division 12, Clinical Psychology, Division 45, Ethnic Minority Issues and Division 52, International Psychology, of the American Psychological Association. She is co-editor of the journal *Women & Therapy*.

The Next Generation: Third Wave Feminist Psychotherapy

CONTENTS

The Next Generation:
Third Wave Feminist Psychotherapy

Ellyn Kaschak

This book is being written early in the new century. Will it be a century that witnesses further gains for feminism and for women, one in which violence and discrimination against women in the United States and in the world are eradicated? Will it be a century where human rights are significantly advanced, if not universally acquired? Or will it be one in which hard-won gains will be lost and the women's movements of the twentieth century eliminated from the history books or relegated to the margins of history?

The last century witnessed the development of a women's movement that made significant gains, but that was lost to the next generation of women. It was eagerly depicted by the written media and in the history books as a small band of odd-looking and frustrated "battle-axes" who sought the vote for women, but who also sought such puritanical objectives as the introduction of prohibition. As they apparently had no fun in their own lives, they sought the identical fate for their male counterparts. Or so the "official" story went.

The girls of my generation might see a photograph or a paragraph about these women in our history books, just enough exposure to convince each of us that we wanted no more information, that any association with the beliefs of these women would result in ridicule at best and a ruined and isolated life at worst. We had no idea that they opposed alcohol as a way to reduce the domestic violence that increased signifi-

[Haworth co-indexing entry note]: "The Next Generation: Third Wave Feminist Psychotherapy." Kaschak, Ellyn. Co-published simultaneously in *Women & Therapy* (The Haworth Press, Inc.) Vol. 23, No. 2, 2001, pp. 1-4; and: *The Next Generation: Third Wave Feminist Psychotherapy* (ed: Ellyn Kaschak) The Haworth Press, Inc., 2001, pp. 1-4. Single or multiple copies of this article are available for a fee from The Haworth Document Delivery Service [1-800-342-9678, 9:00 a.m. - 5:00 p.m. (EST). E-mail address: getinfo@haworthpressinc.com].

1

cantly under its influence. We had no idea that domestic violence had ever been a public or political issue. And we did not really give these first wave feminists a second thought. After all, women had for decades had the vote. Alcohol had remained legal and was a right of adulthood and a rite of passage into adulthood that we looked forward to claiming as soon as we could. If we thought about this group of early feminists at all, we considered their work to be finished. We had only to enjoy the benefits of their rather old-fashioned attitudes and of their toil.

Does this story sound at all familiar? How many times have I heard an almost identical version from my students, from the young women and men who make up my university classes? Or from those young women who trouble to write about my generation's second wave feminism, referred to more and more frequently as '70s feminism, marked forever by the years of its birth rather than those of its life, as if it is incapable of development, as if frozen in time in its infancy.

For young feminists, the most recent metaphorical manifestation dubbed the third wave, the world is a completely different place than it was for the previous generation. Some of the goals of early feminism have been accomplished. We were the first generation permitted entry to the graduate programs and to the professions in significant numbers. Young women take for granted that these avenues are available to them without struggle and without the necessity for political analysis. They find, in many institutions, courses on the Psychology of Women and perhaps even Feminist Therapy. If they are really fortunate, they find mentors and colleagues and much less severe and less overt discrimination than we did. And they find thirty years of theory and practice that has preceded them.

The field is not as we found it. Is that not a cause for celebration, for acknowledgment in every course and in every textbook, not just the explicitly feminist ones? Are feminists not heroes of their culture, deserving plaudits and recognition for the advancement of human rights equaled only perhaps by other liberation movements or revolutions in the name of freedom? History, after all, is nothing more and nothing less than the story of our lives, our dreams, our accomplishments and our failures.

At the same time, there is still much to be done. We are still too far from equality, from safety and from elimination or even reduction of all the personal psychological suffering induced in individual women by constant exposure to the many forms of cultural inequity. We are still too far from the basic respect for women that would have to include respect for feminism and understanding that women's rights are simply basic human rights. There may very well be a different temperament, a different style needed for a different historical and cultural time. The tasks before young feminists are different because of all that we accomplished and did not accomplish and because it is a different world from the one in which we fought for freedom and equality. Yet they need the connection with the previous generation and with each other as much as we do. They need mentors in academia, in the study of psychology and in the practice of psychotherapy.

In this issue, young feminists themselves describe their lives and struggles, speak of the issues that they find important and of the cultural context in which they have come of age. We present dialogues between second and third wave feminists, along with the individual voices of the young feminists themselves.

In their intergenerational analysis, Sharon Horne, Susan Mathews, Pam Detrie, Mary Burke and Becky Cook find that emerging feminists come to their feminism differently as they are in a different cultural context than were second wave feminists. Specifically they face the dilemma of reconciling two different cultural discourses, that of the classroom which tends to credit feminism for many cultural strides and that of the popular media, which portrays feminists negatively. Cindy Bruns and Colleen Trimble also discuss the social and historical context of young women's lives and how they might have been lulled into a false sense that feminism is no longer necessary in this new century. They show that feminism is germane to third wave psychotherapists and then focus on issues of power with a particular emphasis on relational power. Cindy Veldhuis considers power as it has been approached historically with regard to feminist therapy and identifies areas where younger feminist therapists can help continue to define and to clarify this important issue. The authors of these two articles see the issue of power as a central one for young feminist psychotherapists.

Natalie Porter, Dalia Ducker, Holley Ferrel and Laura Helton also present an intergenerational dialogue in which they explore the relationships of feminists of these two generations with a particular focus on the importance of mentoring. Jill Rader offers her perspective on the centrality of the mentoring process in the development of feminist therapists. Lisa Rubin and Carol Nemeroff emphasize the importance of intergenerational dialogue between second and third wave women and give us yet another example of how to begin.

Finally, Norine Johnson presents a novel feminist approach for working with adolescent girls who have not yet been assigned a wave number. In this process, the girl is empowered to become an equal partner with her therapist and in shaping the therapeutic endeavor. This closing article extends the intergenerational theme to the generation that has not yet come of age or come to feminism with the aim of facilitating their strength, self-confidence and emerging partnership.

Implicit in this discussion is a concern with reaching the young women who do not identify themselves as feminists. The media and the larger culture still make "I'm not a feminist . . ." seem a safe haven. In a sense, we have also made it possible to say, "I'm not a feminist, but . . ." by our very accomplishments. Yet there is so much left to be accomplished by feminists and our allies. Finally achieving respect for women must translate into pride in calling oneself a feminist. To that end, I want to both acknowledge and express appreciation to all the women and men of all generations who have had the courage, the pride and the self-respect to call themselves feminists and the strength and determination to practice feminism.

Look It Up Under "F":
Dialogues of Emerging
and Experienced Feminists

Sharon Horne
Susan Mathews
Pam Detrie
Mary Burke
Becky Cook

SUMMARY. This article explores the process of integrating a feminist identity for both experienced and emerging feminists. A qualitative analysis was utilized to identify themes in two group dialogues. The analysis indicated that the era in which experienced feminists were initiated into feminism framed this movement as liberating and empowering, while emerging feminists described a process of initial resistance when encountering feminism. Emerging feminists discussed having to overcome negative media images of feminism before becoming motivated to integrate this identity. Both groups relayed challenges in communicating feminist principles and the practices they used to meet these difficulties. Findings in this article are discussed in relation to the need for a sensitive

Sharon Horne, Susan Mathews, Pam Detrie, Mary Burke, and Becky Cook are affiliated with the Department of Counseling, Educational Psychology and Research at the University of Memphis.

Address correspondence to: Sharon Horne, Department of Counseling, Educational Psychology and Research, The University of Memphis, 100 Educational Building, Memphis, TN 38152 (E-mail: shorne@memphis.edu).

The authors thank Shelby Crump-Jetton for her assistance in transcribing the data.

[Haworth co-indexing entry note]: "Look It Up Under 'F': Dialogues of Emerging and Experienced Feminists." Horne, Sharon et al. Co-published simultaneously in *Women & Therapy* (The Haworth Press, Inc.) Vol. 23, No. 2, 2001, pp. 5-18; and: *The Next Generation: Third Wave Feminist Psychotherapy* (ed: Ellyn Kaschak) The Haworth Press, Inc., 2001, pp. 5-18; Single or multiple copies of this article are available for a fee from The Haworth Document Delivery Service [1-800-342-9678, 9:00 a.m. - 5:00 p.m. (EST). E-mail address: getinfo@haworthpressinc.com].

5

presentation of feminism to young women in classrooms or professional settings. *[Article copies available for a fee from The Haworth Document Delivery Service: 1-800-342-9678. E-mail address: <getinfo@haworthpressinc.com> Website: <http://www.HaworthPress.com> © 2001 by The Haworth Press, Inc. All rights reserved.]*

KEYWORDS. Feminism, feminist identity development, mentoring, women's movement, psychology, therapy

INTRODUCTION

The opportunity for women to informally discuss their experiences, as well as feminist issues and ideas, all but disappeared with the decline of consciousness-raising groups in the early 1980s (Horne, 1999; Kirsh, 1987). Consciousness-raising groups emerged in response to an increasing awareness of women's social and cultural oppression and the inadequacy of traditional psychotherapy to meet their needs. They grew in popularity in the 1960s in the United States (Broverman, Broverman, Clarkson, Rosenkrantz, & Vogel, 1970; Enns, 1993), driven by the belief that women meeting and sharing experiences would offset the effects of sexism and decrease the isolation commonly reported by women. In particular, these groups were rooted in the idea that personal experience is at the very root of social and political change (Horne, 1991).

The effect of women meeting and taking action together as part of the feminist movement is well documented. The successful passage of *Roe v. Wade*, the inclusion of sexual harassment legislature, the Violence Against Women Act, the creation of a national infrastructure of crisis centers for women, as well as increasing numbers of women in the workforce and in the upper echelons of management, are just a few examples of the influence of the feminist movement.

In the mid-1980s, the agenda of women's groups shifted from consciousness-raising to the provision of support for members seeking assistance in coping with particular social and personal issues (e.g., codependency groups, assertiveness training; Kirsh, 1987). For those young women interested in learning more about the women's movement, the opportunities were restricted by the availability of formal education in the form of emerging women's studies programs. Although feminists continued to advance the social and political position of women, the use of the label "feminist" began to fall out of favor among young women (Faludi, 1991). The media increasingly began to portray feminism in a negative light (e.g., Faludi, 1991), often equating it to lesbianism and to female aggression.

Despite the response of many feminist scholars to this backlash, it can be argued that young women today still are in the process of negotiating their relationship to their feminist identities. They are confronted with hostile images of feminism in the mainstream media, yet within the classroom, they often are forced to credit feminism with many social strides. In order to investigate how they reconcile these two different discourses, and to study cross-generational differences, the authors have interviewed two sets of feminists about the development of their feminist identities and the meaning of feminism in their lives. The idea of the study emerged from a bimonthly discussion group of doctoral students discovering feminist psychology and theory. This group of emerging feminists became interested in how experienced feminists would discuss the meaning and impact of feminism on their lives and whether there would be differences between the two groups.

REVIEW OF THE LITERATURE

The women's rights movement has been defined by Ould (1998) as "occurring in waves" of feminist activity. These "waves" of the women's rights movement are based upon differing social and historical contexts that have resulted in women's varying understanding of the meaning of feminism. The first wave is associated with women's suffrage, while the second wave began with Friedan's work entitled *The Feminine Mystique* (1963), in which the rights of women to establish their own careers and to identify themselves within roles other than that of wife and mother were presented. Finally, the current third wave of feminism has been distinguished by its emphasis on factors of oppression other than gender (i.e., race, sexual orientation, socio-economic status, and disability status). This new movement has not yet been "firmly established by a specific event, yet young women are writing and talking about a third wave" (Ould, 1998, p. 146).

Recent literature in the field of psychology has also begun to focus attention on the unique aspects of women's identity development from a feminist perspective (Gilligan, 1982; Jordan, Kaplan, Miller, & Stiver, 1991; Miller, 1986). Specifically, feminist researchers are exploring the ways in which women understand and define themselves within a broad framework of social contexts. Exploration of these sociopolitical and cultural contexts has led to the examination of female identity as defined within a patriarchal society and a corresponding reconstruction of female identity as a feminist identity, including an appreciation of female characteristics and values. Feminist identity has been conceptualized as a developmental process women experience as they encounter sociopolitical influences, such as sexism, and determine the ways in which these forces impact their lives (McNamara & Rickard, 1989).

Downing and Roush (1985) created a model of feminist identity development that explains the process through five stages. In the first stage of the model, passive-acceptance, the women adhere to traditional sex roles, accept the superiority of men, and fail to acknowledge discrimination against women within society. Stage two of the model, revelation, is exemplified by a consciousness-raising experience in which the individual develops anger through a questioning process, resulting in a new understanding of the forces of oppression in her life. The third stage is characterized by embeddedness in female culture. Close affiliations are formed with other like-minded women. These relationships create a safe, woman-friendly environment in which women process feelings of anger and betrayal and receive nurturance and affirmation. In the fourth stage, synthesis, the individual forms a positive feminist identity that integrates the understanding that oppression has an impact on women, with an emphasis on the multiple layers of social oppression. Finally, the fifth stage, active commitment, is a culmination of the previous stages in which the individual channels her feminist identity into activities promoting the creation of social change. The Feminist Identity Development model described by Downing and Roush (1985) suggests that as a woman becomes more aware of patriarchy's oppressive influence on her development, she moves to a more "advanced" level of feminist identity.

Research centered on models of feminist identity development has attempted to establish connections between levels of feminist identity and self-esteem (Rickard, 1987), coping strategies (Dell, 1999), and personal reactions to definitions of feminism (Jackson et al., 1996; Kamen, 1991; and Korman, 1983). Positive associations were established in these research findings between higher levels of feminist identity development and higher levels of self-esteem, problem-solving coping styles, and support for feminist constructs, respectively. To date, the majority of contributions made to understanding the development of a feminist identity have attempted to quantify and describe women's growth within the context of established theoretical models such as that proposed by Downing and Roush (1985), which was adapted from Cross's (1995) model of racial identity development.

In contrast to previous research formats on feminist identity development that have focused on employing theoretical models, such as Downing and Roush's (1985) attempt to define women's experiences, the current qualitative study employed a discovery-oriented approach to explore the experiences of feminists from the participants' personal perspectives. Structured discussions were conducted with two groups of women to investigate the feminist themes emerging within their dialogues. The first group of third wave, "Emerging Feminists" was composed of women coming into their feminist identities through graduate work, while the second group of second wave, "Experienced Feminists" was comprised of women who have engaged in multiple forms of feminist activism for many years.

METHOD

Participants

Emerging Feminists. Four women who have begun to identify as feminists within the last two years of doctoral study in a counseling psychology program were categorized as emerging feminists. These women ranged in age from mid-twenties to mid-forties. They were interviewed in March 2000 for approximately two hours in Memphis, Tennessee. Participants were recruited via membership in the "Power Women Group," a group of doctoral students that meets bimonthly to discuss feminist theories and works with a feminist faculty advisor.

Experienced Feminists. Four women who discovered feminism between the late 1960s and early 1980s were categorized as experienced feminists. These women ranged in age from mid-forties to mid-sixties. They were interviewed on two occasions for approximately an hour and thirty minutes each at the Association of Women in Psychology Conference in Salt Lake City in March 2000. Participants were recruited via e-mail prior to the conference and asked to participate in this study. They were identified as noteworthy feminist scholars and psychologists who had contributed to the field by virtue of their histories of publication, teaching, and practice of feminist psychotherapy.

Data Collection

This study utilized two group interviews. One of the authors, the faculty advisor for the emerging feminists, served as a facilitator for both groups of experienced and emerging feminists. An emerging feminist co-facilitated the interviews of the experienced feminists but acted solely as a participant within the interview of emerging feminists. Transcription of these taped interviews was completed by a graduate student who was separate from the project. When acting as facilitators, the faculty advisor and the emerging feminist took precautions to employ language that was open-ended, to paraphrase close to the language of participants, and to indicate explicitly that they were interested in hearing all of their participants' experiences and had no preconceived ideas of what topics were expected to emerge.

Data Analysis

The data analysis was based upon grounded theory methodology introduced by Glaser and Strauss (1967). This rigorous procedure is an inductive method in which investigators build theory from the intensive analysis of text.

In this study, transcripts of the two interviews were divided consensually by three of the investigators into meaning units (see Merleau-Ponty, 1962; Giorgi, 1970), segments of text defined by the presence of only one core idea. In accordance with grounded theory, these units were organized using the process of constant comparison and initial categories were formed, reflecting similarities between meaning units. The initial categories were labeled in language grounded in the transcripts and these labels were then grouped into higher-order categories to form a hierarchical structure. The authors kept a log throughout the process of analysis in an attempt to "bracket" their experiences so that they wouldn't influence the structuring of the data hierarchy. These memos were reflected upon once the data categorization process was complete and used to enrich the discussion of findings.

The authors adapted the process of grounded theory to better suit the procedure to the structure of the group interviews. Although the data collection could not be guided by theoretical sampling, the investigators did attempt to include participants who were varied by age, class, race and forms of employment within these groups. Also, in a traditional method, based upon individual interviews, investigators stopped interviewing once they found that no new categories were being suggested by incoming data. In the present study, only one interview was conducted with each group and so the termination of data collection could not be signaled by saturation. The investigators did note, however, that no new categories seemed to be forthcoming in the latter half of each interview analysis, suggestive of saturation

Following the interviews, the emerging feminists were provided with the transcripts and asked for their reflections on accuracy and content. This process provided them with an opportunity to clarify their statements regarding the interview.

RESULTS

This analysis of the transcript of the emerging feminist interview generated 133 meaning units that were organized into 22 initial categories. The analysis of the experienced feminist interview yielded 191 meaning units, which were organized into 31 initial categories. The difference in numbers of meaning units and hierarchies might be suggestive of the greater complexity of experienced feminists' understanding of feminism and their longer life experience with feminism. Both hierarchies had three levels of categorization. For the purpose of concision, the two higher-order categories will be discussed below.

Emerging Feminists

The highest-order categories in this analysis were: Initiation into Feminism, Integration of Feminist Identity, and Realization of Feminist Subtexts. In order to address their initiation into feminism, the participants described a variety of situations through which they first became exposed to feminist thought. Women stated that they lacked an understanding of feminism and felt that their limited exposure to feminism was intimidating due to the "radical" and negative images portrayed in the media. Emerging feminists discussed coming into their feminism through exposure to concepts in their doctoral graduate training. Namely, the participants expressed that once they were exposed to a definition of feminism that was straightforward (i.e., feminists promote equality for women) it could not be dismissed. Once these women began to incorporate feminist constructs into their thinking, they described their emerging feminist awareness as a validating experience that provided a "label" for a core sense of feminism that had been present "all along."

As well this learning provided a more expansive vocabulary and alternative way of seeing the world. These women reported that their initiation into feminism was positive as it "sparked a fire" of interest and excitement in their willingness to learn, and yet it also highlighted the visibility of oppression and sexism in their daily lives. Finally, the emerging feminists addressed the abstract nature of feminism and their difficulty making contact with other feminists. One woman described her experience, "I knew that feminism was something that I believed in but it was so hard to see how I could be a part of it. It seemed like something so far away from me. Well, how do I do that? Is this something I can look up in the phone book?" As they could not locate feminist organizations under "F" in the phone book, it was difficult for these women to identify a way of making entry into meaningful feminist activism.

Emerging feminists addressed their expression and integration of feminist identities primarily in the context of their clinical practice of psychology. Also, these women discussed the gradual development of their multiple identities (i.e., feminist, lesbian, and therapist), that had become integrated and inseparable within their perception of themselves. In addition, emerging feminists explored the importance of considering the context of their environment prior to expressing feminist beliefs that may be perceived as "radical," in an attempt to maintain their audience. Further, emerging feminists expressed concern about viewing activism as an all-or-nothing dichotomy, lacking sensitivity to the multiple forms of activism in their daily personal and professional interactions. Finally, these women also considered the "risks" associated with publicly expressing their feminist beliefs in multiple contexts (i.e., professional settings or familial relationships). They wrestled with the "price" exacted by being outspoken about their feminist beliefs, but recognized the alternative costs of maintaining silence.

Three themes surfaced in the emerging feminists' discussion that related their realization of feminist subtexts. First, the women recognized that it is impossible to fulfill the societal expectations that they should strive to "have it all" in reference to a career outside of the home, as well as a marriage and children. The participants felt that the myth of "having it all" places an onus upon women to adjust their personal desires to meet the constraints of their environment. The expectations placed upon modern women were thought to pathologize individual women's struggle with balancing work and family and hence to undermine the motivation for social organization to promote change. Secondly, the emerging feminists recognized that they were always given the message that they could do or be "anything" they desired (i.e., professionally). However, these women also recognized that within this supportive message was a strong "but," which served as a transition to the list of limitations that would inevitably follow. Namely, these women described messages such as: "You can do anything you want to do, but you must also get married and have a family." Finally, the emerging feminists described several examples in which their adherence to and discussion of feminist principles placed them "outside their family boxes," thereby resulting in conflict or feelings of discomfort.

Experienced Feminists

The highest-order categories in this analysis were: Initiation into Feminism, Gifts of Feminism: What the Meaning of Feminism Is All About, and the Transition and Nuances of Feminist Identity. Experienced feminists addressed their initiation into feminism in two main movements. Specifically, the women differentiated a sense of coming into feminism from early in life as opposed to gaining an awareness of feminist thought through an "awakening" process. The experienced feminists referenced several sources through which they gained their exposure to feminist principles. Namely, the women described multiple experiences surrounding their coming into feminism through pursuing graduate education, exploring written works addressing feminist constructs, and interacting with and receiving guidance from feminist role models and mentors. In addition, the experienced feminists addressed the ways in which significant historical movements and cultural influences had an impact on their awareness of feminism. The women addressed the significant influence of the Human Rights, Civil Rights, Womanist, and Women's movements, as well as their own cultural backgrounds (for example, African-American upbringing, Southern traditional values) on their initiation into feminism.

The experienced feminists' discussion of the "gifts of feminism" described the excitement associated with the empowering aspects of feminism in their lives. The women stated that finding feminism provided them with a context and label that validated the experiences of women in general, as well as each participants' experiences individually. The experienced feminists addressed feminism as a radical idea during the 1970s, during which time feminism was a new way of looking at the world and was often stereotyped with lesbianism. In addition, the women described feminism as a political movement in which many forms of activism exist. Specifically, the women referred to feminism on a continuum from an initially liberal to emerging radical practice. The experienced feminists also discussed the transition and nuances associated with the change in feminist expression. A significant emphasis of the women's discussion focused on power, class, and culture within the context of a growing emphasis on radical, multicultural, and global feminism. The experienced feminists expressed an awareness that although the meaning of the word "feminism" has remained consistent over time, the use of the word "feminist" has become "scary" and often brings negative consequences. As one participant stated, "To be a feminist in this world today is to be revolutionary." Therefore, within many interactions, the experienced feminists have begun to utilize the constructs of feminism without applying the label of feminism itself, depending upon the context and their audiences. In addition, the experienced feminists discussed the importance of expressing their "voices, energies, and resilience" by engaging in activism in many forms. The women recognized that discriminatory practices have consistently become more subtle over time, which has resulted in a need for more "sophisticated" forms of feminist activism. Finally, the experienced feminists expressed the view that feminist movements are numerous and "alive," despite the fact that many of the grassroots women's organizations are not organized in a traditional corporate structure. These women stress the importance of acknowledging the many gifts of feminism, particularly in light of the incorporation of feminist principles, ideologies, theories, and practices into standard psychological practices.

DISCUSSION

The development of a feminist identity appears to have differed remarkably between the two groups of experienced feminists and emerging feminists. While experienced feminists talked about the excitement of "awakening" into feminism during a time of heightened interest in human rights and Civil Rights, the emerging feminists discussed their initial exposure to feminism as intimidating, with negative images of "bra-burning radicals." For the experienced feminists, there was a women's movement already in place or, at the very least, evolving, and the participants shared their experiences of joining groups of women for mutual support, finding role models and mentors, and reading feminist works, all of which helped participants to solidify a feminist identity. In contrast, emerging feminists spoke of their frustration at not having any formal exposure to feminism during their undergraduate careers and feeling as if they had no understanding of feminism that fit with their vision of themselves until much further into their education.

These findings support recent work (Enns, 1993; Horne, 1999; Kirsch, 1987) that suggests that for emerging feminists, consciousness-raising groups and active movements such as the women's movement, the Civil Rights movement, and the human rights movement, have not been central in the foundation of their feminist identities. While the emerging feminists discussed their burgeoning activism as exciting or "having sparked a fire," they also were quick to share their initial distrust of feminism. Their self-described resistance could not be maintained, however, once provided with a more complete exposure to the central tenets of feminism. These women credited their doctoral training with their primary exposure to feminism and emphasized their relationships with peers and colleagues as instrumental in cementing their feminist identities.

Both sets of participants emphasized that for feminist principles to be most effective, they should be expressed with the consideration of context and adaptation to their social environment. The women explained that they had developed styles of "coming out" as feminists depending on the situation, with the intention of not "losing" the person by appearing too radical. Both sets used a variety of subversive means to maintain the positive meanings of feminism, including employing questioning techniques that highlighted power inequalities, teaching constructs without employing the label of feminism, and using feminist language to describe oppression, sexism, and social inequalities. Both groups recognized that the use of the feminist label often invoked negative consequences.

Emerging feminists also differed from experienced feminists in terms of the gender role messages they received. While experienced feminists talked about the fact that they were raised primarily with strong expectations of adherence to traditional gender roles, emerging feminists discussed receiving messages that they "could do anything and be anyone" but only as long as "it included marriage and mothering." Along with this, emerging feminists talked about growing up with the message of "women should be able to have it all," which covertly meant women should be able to balance successfully a career and family while men were applauded for "helping out."

In comparison with the experienced women, emerging feminists described a more active process of putting their ideals into action with family and stepping outside of the box to test their boundaries. This engagement makes sense given where these women are in their professional and personal development. The experiences of these emerging feminist women call into question the relevance of the feminist identity development model of Downing and Roush (1985), particularly the passive acceptance stage in which there is an acceptance of traditional sex roles, and the belief in the superiority of men. The emerging feminists appeared not to have entered a stage of passive acceptance; rather they were raised to believe that traditional sex roles were no longer applicable and would not hinder their career and family aspirations.

Both emerging and experienced feminists emphasized that activism takes many forms. Experienced feminists stressed that as discriminatory practices have become more subtle, feminism has become more sophisticated. Therefore, it is encouraging that both groups seemed to recognize the importance of activism being expressed one-on-one, collectively, and globally. At the same time, the experienced feminists expressed feeling bittersweet that feminist principles, theories, and practices often are incorporated into standard psychological practices without acknowledgment.

The themes that evolved from the interview with emerging feminists highlight some important considerations for educators and therapists working with young women. It is clear from their discussions that many young women will hold conflictual and inaccurate beliefs about feminism and will have been exposed to negative views of feminism. Therefore, it may be important in initial discussions of feminism to make clear the definitions and constructs of feminism. Because young women have fewer venues for discussion of feminist ideas than their experienced feminist colleagues, they may have pressing needs for group dialogues and discussions as well as feminist mentoring relationships. Educators, wishing to make explicit that oppression of women continues to thrive, may need to demonstrate the systematic and subtle forces of discrimination and abuses of power since many young women fail to see oppression given the successful strides of feminism in the past thirty years. Finally, feminists should "come out" with a capital "F" and when the context doesn't lend itself safely to identifying with the label, feminists should find ways to continue to employ the constructs.

REFERENCES

Broverman, I., Broverman, D., Clarkson, F., Rosenkrantz, P., & Vogel, S. (1970). Sex role stereotypes and clinical judgments of mental health. *Journal of Consulting Psychology, 34*, 1-7.

Cross, W. E., Jr. (1995). The psychology of Nigresence: Revising the Cross model. In J. G. Ponterotto, J. M. Casas, L. A. Suzuki, and C. M. Alexander (Eds.), *Handbook of Multicultural Counseling*, Thousand Oaks, CA: Sage, pp. 93-122.

Dell, G. M. (1999). Female mental health professionals' feminist identity development, gender-role attitudes, and coping styles. *Dissertation Abstracts International, 60 (2A).*

Downing, N. E., & Roush, K. L. (1985). From passive acceptance to active commitment: A model of feminist identity development for women. *The Counseling Psychologist, 13*, 695-709.

Enns, C. Z. (1993). Twenty years of feminist counseling and therapy: From naming biases to implementing multifaceted practice. *The Counseling Psychologist, 21* (1), 3-87.

Faludi, S. (1991). *Backlash: The undeclared war against American women.* New York: Anchor Books.

Friedan, B. (1963). *The feminine mystique.* New York: Dell Publishing Co., Inc.

Gilligan, C. (1982). *In a different voice: Psychological theory and women's development.* Cambridge, MA: Harvard University Press.

Giorigi, A. (1970). *Psychology as a human science: A phenomenological approach.* New York: Harper & Row.

Glaser, B. J., & Strauss, A. (1967). *The discovery of grounded theory: Strategies for qualitative research.* Chicago IL: Aldine.

Home, A. (1991). Mobilizing women's strengths for social change: The group connection. *Social Work with Groups, 14*, 153-173.

Horne, S. (1999). From coping to creating change: The evolution of women's groups. *Journal of Specialists in Group Work, 43*, 333-335.

Jackson, L. A., Fleury, R. E., & Lewandowski, D. A. (1996). Feminism: Definitions, support, and correlates of support among female and male college students. *Sex Roles, 34* (9/10), 687-693.

Jordan, J. V. (1985). The meaning of mutuality. In J. V. Jordon, A. G. Kaplan, J. B. Miller, I. P. Silver, & J. Surrey (Eds.), *Women's growth in connection: Writings from the Stone Center* (pp. 81-96). New York, NY: Guilford Press.

Kamen, P. (1991). *Feminist fatale: Voices from the "twentysomething" generation explore the future of the "Women's Movement."* New York: Donald I. Fine, Inc.

Kirsh, B. (1987). Consciousness raising and self-help groups. In C. Brody (Ed.), *Women's therapy groups: Paradigms of feminist treatment* (pp. 43-54). New York: Springer Publishing Company.

Korman, S. K. (1983). The feminist-familial influences on adherence to ideology and commitment to a self-perception. *Family Relations, 32*, 431-439.

McNamara, K., & Rickard, K. M. (1989). Feminist identity development: Implications for feminist therapy with women. *Journal of Counseling and Development, 68*, 184-189.

Merleau-Ponty, M. (1962). *Phenomenology of perception* (Colin Smith, Trans). London and New York: Routledge.

Miller, J. B. (1976). *Toward a new psychology of women.* Boston: Beacon Press.

Miller, J. B. (1988). Connections, disconnections and violations. *Work in Progress, No. 33.* Wellesley, MA: Stone Center Working Paper Series.

Ould, P. J. (1998). Women and sociology: How the structure of society affects women. In D. M. Ashcraft (Ed.), *Women's work: A survey of scholarship by and about women* (pp. 135-165). Binghamton, NY: Harrington Park Press.

Rickard, K. (1987, March). *A model of feminist identity development.* Association for Women in Psychology, Denver, Colorado.

Surry, J. L. (1983). The self-in-relation: A theory of women's development. In J. V. Jordon, A. G. Kaplan, J. B. Miller, I. P. Silver, & J. Surrey (Eds.), *Women's growth in connection: Writings from the Stone Center* (pp. 51-66). New York, NY: Guilford Press.

Worrell, J., & Remer, P. (1992). *Feminist perspectives in therapy: An empowerment model for women.* West Sussex, England: John Whiley & Sons.

Rising Tide:
Taking Our Place
as Young Feminist Psychologists

Cindy M. Bruns
Colleen Trimble

SUMMARY. Many wonder what the third wave of feminism will bring
ashore as young feminists begin taking their place in various aspects of
professional psychology. We begin by examining how the developmental context of young feminists can prevent us from bringing the riches of
previous generations into our own work. We also examine how our context allows us to make unique contributions in feminism. We will discuss
our attempts to claim a notion of power that is neither hierarchical nor
egalitarian, but relational. Finally, we will end by considering the implications of relational power for the third wave and feminist psychology. *[Article copies available for a fee from The Haworth Document Delivery
Service: 1-800-342-9678. E-mail address: <getinfo@haworthpressinc.com>
Website: <http://www.HaworthPress.com> © 2001 by The Haworth Press, Inc.
All rights reserved.]*

Cindy M. Bruns, MA, and Colleen Trimble, MA, are currently psychology interns
at the Texas Woman's University Counseling Center (TWUCC).

Cindy is a doctoral candidate at the California School of Professional Psychology,
Alameda campus, at Alliant University.

Colleen is a doctoral candidate at the Chicago School of Professional Psychology.

Address correspondence to: Cindy M. Bruns, Denton County Friends of the Family,
P.O. Box 640, Denton, TX 76202-0640 (E-mail: cindymbruns@sprintmail.com).

The authors wish to thank the training committee at TWUCC for their support and encouragement for writing this article. They also wish to thank Christianne McKee and
Pamela Birrell for their thoughtful dialogues about the nature of power and for their edito-
rial comments.

[Haworth co-indexing entry note]: "Rising Tide: Taking Our Place as Young Feminist Psychologists."
Bruns, Cindy M., and Colleen Trimble. Co-published simultaneously in *Women & Therapy* (The Haworth
Press, Inc.) Vol. 23, No. 2, 2001, pp. 19-36; and: *The Next Generation: Third Wave Feminist Psychotherapy*
(ed: Ellyn Kaschak) The Haworth Press, Inc., 2001, pp. 19-36. Single or multiple copies of this article are
available for a fee from The Haworth Document Delivery Service [1-800-342-9678, 9:00 a.m. - 5:00 p.m.
(EST). E-mail address: getinfo@haworthpressinc.com].

KEYWORDS. Third wave feminism, power, young feminists, diversity

The dawning of the 21st century is a time of significant change for all of society. The realm of feminist psychology is not immune to the currents of change. In fact, the rising tide bringing forth the third wave of feminists is breaking on the shore of psychology. Many wonder what this wave will bring ashore as young feminists begin to take their place in various aspects of the profession. Others, perhaps, wonder if this new wave will wash from the shore all traces of the first and second waves. To understand the offerings and struggles of this generation, one must examine the effects of the context into which we were born, raised, and trained. In particular, our context is one in which there is some built-in gender privilege and decreased experiences of overt sexism, and a deeper and broader incorporation of all types of diversity into our consciousness, and in which the postmodern movement has challenged notions of reality and truth at fundamental levels. As much as others must understand the context of the third wave, young feminists must recognize and mine the rich minerals left in the wake of prior waves, recognizing the contributions of our foremothers, feminist and those who historically have felt marginalized from the feminist movement, and finding a way to "pay homage to, while moving away from, previous feminist formulations" (Alliaume, 1998).

This article will begin by examining the ways in which the developmental context of young feminists can prevent this generation from bringing the riches of previous generations into our own work. These include: (a) the loss of subversive stories from young feminists' memories (Fletcher, 1999), (b) the tendency to believe we are the end product of the feminist fight rather than part of a continuing process and disregard the political activism aspects of feminist psychology, and (c) the tendency to be blind to the undertow of the backlash.

Coming into our own as feminists within a context of some privilege and a greater understanding of diverse contextual issues, while producing difficulties, also has allowed third wave feminists to reformulate some important concepts in the field of psychology. In this article, we will consider one of these concepts: the meaning of power. We will discuss ways young feminists are attempting to claim a notion of power that is neither hierarchical nor egalitarian. We will deconstruct these traditional conceptualizations of power and propose relational power as an alternative method for performing power. Finally, we will end by considering the implications of relational power for: (a) dialogues between diverse members of the feminist community, including those traditionally marginalized by and alienated from feminism; (b) the professional development of young feminists; (c) working with clients and colleagues; and (d) restoring to the third wave the political activism needed to stem the tide of the backlash.

A final note is important before addressing the issues with which this article is concerned. As stated above, understanding the contextual issues that helped shape third wave feminists is important to understanding their point of view and work in the field of psychology. Similarly, our embedded contexts, as authors of this article, are important to an understanding of the views we will articulate. Many of our contexts are discussed via our exploration of the general context of young feminists, as we both began life in the late 1960s or early 1970s. However, contexts that may remain hidden include our racial and ethnic privilege by virtue of being of Euro-American descent, economic privilege through inclusion in the middle class, and, for one of the authors, heterosexual privilege. As various types of social privileging interact to either increase or decrease overall status, we recognize our experience of decreased sexism is due, in part, to the privilege we have been granted by virtue of contexts other than gender. In addition, our graduate training in psychology has occurred in professional schools. Professional schools, in some ways, stand outside traditional academic environs, allowing our development to include a wider exposure to, training in, and dialogue about cultural issues than our colleagues in more traditional training settings. This context also colors our perceptions of the field of psychology and its direction for the future. With these contextual issues in mind, we now turn to the broader social context whose waxing helped bring about the third wave of feminism.

FOLLOWING THE SECOND WAVE OUT TO SEA

Lost at Sea: The Birth of Feminism's Next Generation

The context of the world into which we were born has contributed undeniably to who we are as we enter the field of Psychology. We are "Generation X." In our earliest years, those around us breathed a sigh of relief as they witnessed the end of the Vietnam War. This feeling of peace, however, was short-lived and soon replaced by growing horror at the thought of nuclear destruction, either at the hands of the vilified Russians, or, as witnessed by such accidents as Three Mile Island, at our own hands. The perception of this threat was lessened significantly some years later as we cheered on the fall of the Berlin Wall and the more extensive fall of Communism in Eastern Europe. We saw ourselves as part of an aggressive world power that would not hesitate to risk the lives of U.S. soldiers, as well as soldiers and civilians of many other countries, to reinforce this status.

We spent the majority of our youth under the leadership of Reagan and Bush and felt the harsh effects of Reaganomics. At a time when materialism and greed were growing exponentially, we grew up with more and more people having less and less money and even higher-income households needing dual incomes. We witnessed many more divorces and single-parent homes. We saw ourselves or our classmates becoming what would be termed "latchkey kids," sustained by an ever-growing diet of television and fast food. We found ourselves being promised a successful future if we obtained a college degree, only to graduate into the deepest economic recession of recent years. Even now, we are again on the verge of graduation into a field that is struggling to support its current members, much less the increasing number of budding psychologists.

This persistent erosion in our lives of those ideals and beliefs which we held dear contrasted greatly with our parents' generation, who gained some comfort by being able to believe there was an undeniable reality, that what they knew to be the truth was, in fact, the Truth. Instead, our lives started out about the time of Watergate, when President Nixon lied to the people of the country on television. He would turn out to be the first of many supposed role models we would witness committing crimes and labeling something the truth, only later to be exposed as fraud. We are a generation of people who are not only *not* surprised when those in power intentionally mislead us, but, in fact, expect them to do so. It follows that we grew up questioning those in authority and what they claimed to be truth, as well as questioning ourselves and challenging our own assumptions and beliefs about what we saw as the truth. This made us willing students of the philosophical movement postmodernism, in which alternatives to what is presented as the Truth are explored and expected. We have grown up, in fact, in a postmodern era, a time in which less was assumed and assured and more was questioned and disbelieved.

Although the state of the world has led us to become part of a cynical and sometimes pessimistic generation, our ideas about women and their place in society have been much more hope-inspiring and, in fact, perhaps one of the few things we took for granted. We were born into a time when women could be seen in a greater number of roles than at any previous time. We saw women working in a broad range of fields. We saw women on television who were assertive, opinionated and strong. We saw women anchoring the evening news. We saw women on the Supreme Court and in a variety of political positions. We saw a woman run for vice president. We saw women as part of space shuttle crews. We looked all around us and saw women who we not only aspired to be, but who we unquestioningly believed that we could be.

Feminism: Calming the Waters of Discontent

The women we saw in the world around us led us to make assumptions about ourselves as women and our place in society. Perhaps, unlike other assumptions with which we grew up, we did not question those that maintained our privilege and, through our acceptance, avoided calling into question our own status. These assumptions lulled us into believing that all women had always been just as we saw them now. Significant events and struggles within the women's movement happened either years before we were born or when we were very young. We have vague memories of monumental events which happened when we were young, and have been told stories about "the way things used to be." These narratives, however, can all too easily become stories and memories without meaning. As a result, we have incorporated the effects of these events into our lives without fully understanding or appreciating the historical process that gave us the opportunities we now have.

As relatively privileged young girls, we grew up believing that we could truly do whatever we wanted. Further, we were blinded to or confused by those girls of color or other minority status who, experiencing a different truth, did not have this same perception. We did not see ourselves as limited to the domestic sphere and, until more recently, came close to discrediting this as a possibility altogether. We believed that if we worked hard and stayed in school, we could eventually become successful in the world of work. Although some fields and majors were still populated primarily by males, we could not imagine a world where women were not welcomed with open arms into higher education. We even saw military schools, the last bastions of good old boy education, be forced to open their doors to female students. We could take classes in Women's Studies and hear about the contributions of women within other fields. We believed that we could succeed in whichever occupational field most interested us. We had no memory of a time before the women's movement fought for equal access to education and employment and equal pay.

We believed ourselves to be in control of our own bodies. We were not old enough to be aware of the significant rights gained by *Roe v. Wade* in 1973. Even in the recent years of threats to this right, we found it difficult to fathom a world where abortion would be illegal. We could not even imagine a time where birth control was not readily accessible, at least to those with economic privilege, much less illegal. Although we were well aware of the horrifying prevalence of violence against women and children, we could not remember a time when women and children were property of men to be treated as they pleased. We have little memory of the time before sexual abuse and rape were recognized as the violent crimes that they are. It is all too easy to forget about the long, hard fight that so many women fought to make it possible for us to grow up with these assumptions.

In the field of psychology it has been relatively easy to continue this trend of optimistic assumptions about ourselves as women and about women within the field as a whole. Significant gains had already been made within the field, which we could all too easily take for granted. Homosexuality as a mental illness had been taken out of the DSM years before and the APA had officially denounced "conversion therapy." The need to consider the diverse contexts from which clients come had been recognized as imperative to ethical treatment (Feminist Therapy Institute, 1987). Freud's ideas about gender and women had long been disputed and "penis envy" was presented as almost laughable. Phyllis Chesler's groundbreaking book *Women and Madness* (1972) already had exposed the deeply gender-biased beliefs about the mental health of women. The Brovermans' study (1970) documenting sex-role stereotyping amongst psychologists had been rediscovered and its indisputable negative consequences on female clients recognized. Jean Baker Miller and the Stone Center had already presented its theories about women's development within relation to others, challenging the traditionally held beliefs of women's "dependency" as indicative of a lack of mental health (Miller, 1976). The Psychology of Women and Women's Mental Health were both names of popular classes as well as topics of ongoing discussions within other more traditional classes. Carol Gilligan's theory about moral development (Gilligan, 1982) was presented in almost the same breath as Kohlberg's. Finally, we entered the field at a time when feminist therapy was, if not readily accepted as "just good therapy," at least not a new concept which we felt responsible to defend.

Having the privilege to grow up as women in a world where such gains had already been realized, we were able to feel as if our lives, our existence and our experience as women truly mattered. Further, we easily could be fooled into thinking not only that others also believed our experience as women mattered, but that it had always been this way. Although we may have been taught there historically were times in which women did not have the rights that we currently hold, we found it difficult to truly integrate the experience of women as a group who have been discounted, silenced and deeply oppressed. The assumptions we feel entitled to make as women today without acknowledging the reality of the past lead to an erasure of "subversive stories" from our memories (Fletcher, 1999). We become isolated as a group of women instead of seeing ourselves as situated within the history of women. We forget the ideas and beliefs about women we hold to be self-evident were all too recently, and with many groups of multiply oppressed women, still are, "subversive stories . . . personal accounts of members of a marginalized group whose voice has been silenced and whose experience has not been counted as knowledge" (Fletcher, 1999, p. 22). We no longer recognize our experience as a view of reality highly contradictory with and resistant of the dominant group belief, but, instead, as reality itself, and ourselves, as part of the dominant group.

Only a Ripple upon Still Waters

At the same time that our vision of women in the world around us gives us strength, the assumptions we make about ourselves as females appear to threaten our ability to provide this strength to future generations of women. The many assumptions discussed above cause us to be unable to claim and integrate our history. The loss of an integrated memory of what it took to get us here may lead to an ultimate assumption that we, as women today, are the end product of the feminist movement and not simply one of many waves in the process.

Unlike the first and second waves of feminists, we do not as clearly see ourselves called to action. We are not part of a large, distinct activist movement as was the first wave's suffrage movement or the second wave's struggle for equal rights. We do not, for the most part, look around us and become outraged at the current state of affairs for women. We do not have laws that prevent us from voting or owning property. We do not have societal norms keeping us from working. Although we are still a far distance from equal rights for all, the progress made towards equality, particularly for white professional women, can lead us to believe there is nothing much left for us to do. We feel free to continue surfing the wave, enjoying the benefits of those who came before us and feeling thankful we do not have such big battles to fight.

Unlike our foremothers, we were not introduced to the idea of feminism through our own outrage at our lack of rights or deep dissatisfaction with our role in society. Instead, we were exposed to feminism much more academically and theoretically. We heard about it in school, discussed it with other women, noted its relevance in our lives, but did not find ourselves fiercely in need of it as did our predecessors. We did not feel the need to participate in consciousness-raising groups as did feminists in the '60s and '70s; instead, we felt our consciousness already had been raised. We read

The Feminist Mystique (Friedan, 1963) and thought "of course" instead of having the dramatic revelation women before us had experienced upon reading it. We did not see any of this as life changing. Instead, it was simply representative of our lives as they were, with gains toward equality achieved, discrimination widely recognized, and a few still "unenlightened" people who were hardly worth our time. Unlike those before us who were willing to fight for their rights, we have come to believe we should not have to fight.

This trend toward locating feminism within the academic environment has had significant consequences. On the one hand, it has helped to develop and legitimize feminist theory and praxis. Therefore, feminist therapy is no longer seen, in most circles, as an alternative or fringe way of conceptualizing therapy. However, by concentrating the development of feminist therapy and, further, feminism within academia, we risk moving away from the experiential and political activism nature of feminism. As stated by Alfonso and Trigilio (1997), it is concerning to think third wave feminism "may be nothing more than academic discourse about discourse, instead of thinking that arises out of and is closely associated with the social and political problems ordinary women face." It is difficult, if not impossible, to be called to political action when primarily hearing feminism presented in "difficult, specialized, jargonistic language . . . accessible only to the most highly educated" (Alfonso & Trigilio, 1997).

Within feminism as a movement, even as we recognized much-needed changes, we saw these very changes already taking place before our eyes. We grew up knowing earlier stages of the women's movement had been exclusionary toward women from diverse backgrounds. As we learned about the Feminist Mystique, we recognized it targeted upper middle class, college educated, white women who had the privilege to be bored with leisure time, and was not representative of women as a whole. We have seen the importance of diverse membership within the feminist movement and relish the addition of women from different ethnic and racial backgrounds, different socioeconomic classes, lesbian and bisexual women and women of different abilities. The integration of diversity within the women's movement, therefore, can seem accomplished and not something for which we need to continue to work.

Watch Out! Strong Undertow–Swimming May Be Deadly

The interaction of our sense of privilege and the belief we are both the end product of political feminism and the future of academic feminism potentially can blind some feminists of the third wave to the gathering storm of patriarchal backlash. There is a sense, perhaps rightly so, that the war has been won and the current skirmishes, begun by an "unenlightened" few, do not require much attention. In its most extreme, one can picture third wave feminists wrapped in the warmth of security and entitlement, sitting on the beach appreciating the beauty of the rising tide, blind to the storm of backlash about to break over the coast. An example of our blindness is the failure of young feminists–especially young, White, middle-class feminists–to recognize the co-opting of "backlash" and "reverse discrimination" by the patriarchy and their association with the men's movement, anti-feminism, and White supremacy. Our failure to realize the implications of such word theft left young feminists shocked and amazed when affirmative action was first overturned and abortion rights challenged. Many from our generation tend to assume any "reasonable person" (i.e., most of the United States) sees things from our perspective. White supremacy, pro-life, family values, False Memory Syndrome, and fathers' rights groups, while viewed with some fear and trepidation, also are viewed as fringe groups incapable of ever really rising to power again. It is as if our generation equates, at least in our own minds, "reasonable person" with "reasonable woman" and third wave feminists are the definition of reasonableness. Our vision of ourselves as feminists with power and privilege in society is the alternate side of the coin that also contains our blindness to the backlash. Recognizing the connection between these two aspects of our existence as the third wave can restore and broaden our vision. The key to our awakening appears to be a deeper and fuller understanding of power, as our current conceptualizations leave this generation blind and politically inert. Yet, paradoxically, the very context that rendered us so passive also contains the roots of our activism when viewed through a different lens.

GATHERING POWER OF THE WAVE

From its inception, the feminist movement has been concerned with power: who has it, how to get it, and what to do with it once we have it. At least within the context of gender analysis, feminists historically have accurately identified who possesses power and devised effective means for claiming this power as their own. Where feminists of previous generations seem to have faltered is in articulating what, once it is won, women should do with power. The second wave perhaps embodies this struggle most clearly. While winning significant battles supporting the rights of women and adding women's voices to the psychological discourse, i.e., gaining power, feminists simultaneously denied power differentials existed, at least between women (Josefowitz Siegel & Larsen, 1990; Lerman & Rigby, 1990). It is as if, after identifying so clearly the abuses and damage inflicted by the hierarchical, power-over approach of the patriarchy, feminism collectively said "not that!" and attempted to repudiate all differentials by turning to egalitarianism. While we acknowledge egalitarianism properly defined does not necessarily imply the absence of power differentials (Brown, 1994), the general *zeitgeist* of "egalitarian means equal" suggests a discomfort with having and using power.

Offered the choice of hierarchical or egalitarian modes of power by the patriarchy and our foremothers respectively, the question facing young feminist psychologists is how are we to perform power in our generation? This question can be raised only from a place of (partially) institutionalized power, for which we are indebted to previous waves of feminism; from our incorporation of non-Western values, for which we are indebted to our sisters of color; and by the situating of feminist thought in academic and postmodern contexts (Alfonso & Trigilio, 1997). The question of how we are to perform power, although presented as an either/or proposition, finds meaning only as a dialectic between these two historical forms of power, from which a third alternative may emerge.

Generally defined, power is the ability or capacity to produce a change, usually in another person or in the larger environment (Miller, 1987; Loomer, 1976). Hierarchical and egalitarian perspectives differ with respect to how they effect change, but share this underlying definition. Hierarchical approaches to power are associated with unilateral, overt expressions of strength, force, control, and authority, whereas egalitarian approaches are associated with collective sharing, nurturing, discussion, and process. Hierarchical power tends to elicit submissiveness, compliance, and covert resistance from those who are the focus of change, while egalitarian power tends to encourage direct expressions of personal experience, an equal exchange of ideas, and value for the collective good. In their extremes, acts of war and Consciousness Raising groups exemplify these two approaches to the exercise of power.

Casting hierarchical and egalitarian power in this light hides the fact that both are rooted in an economic model of power. By economic we do not mean simply direct and indirect financial resources, although socioeconomic status plays an important role in the construal of power for both approaches. Rather, we contend both types of power have at root an unarticulated belief that power is a fixed commodity and increases in power by one lead to decreases in power by another. By definition, hierarchy arranges people in a graded series based on the possession of some attribute (*The American Heritage Dictionary*, 1983), in this case power. For a hierarchy to exist some people must have more and some people must have less. Egalitarian approaches advocate equality for all, implying everyone has the same ability to produce a change in others and an equal division of power. "Equal division," in turn, implies there is a finite amount of power shared among everyone and those with more initial power must share (give away) some of their power so that everyone can be "empowered" to be equals. In this light, egalitarianism is simply a kinder, gentler hierarchy, embarrassed at being a hierarchy, leading to the denial of extant power differentials among its members through an investment in sharing and a focus on commonality of experience. Denial of hierarchy and economics in the construction of egalitarianism creates the conditions for the movement to assume a universality of women's experience, thereby discounting the narratives of women of color, economically disadvantaged women, older women, lesbian women, and women with disabilities. Acknowledging oppression and privilege based on factors other than gender would expose the hierarchy within egalitarianism as well as its, albeit unintended, roots in patriarchal constructions of power.

The feminist movement was soundly called to task for its silencing of subversive narratives (see Kanuha, 1990, for a review). In response, feminist psychology has moved toward a greater incorporation of diverse narratives and experiences, a broadened definition of its areas of concern, and a considered acknowledgment of and response to power differentials (Feminist Therapy Institute, 1990; Fletcher, 1999, 1997; Kanuha, 1990). As important as these changes are, they fail to question the basic definition of power and, as such, are unable to develop a construction of power that does not ultimately draw its sustenance from the waters of patriarchy. We believe until such questioning of fundamental assumptions occurs, feminists will be uncomfortable with the notion of power. Even the most well-intentioned egalitarianism continues to be in some ways a unilateral exercise of power, even if the change one seeks to produce is an increase in another's power. Empowerment in this context runs the risk of being just as maternalistic as the hierarchical model is paternalistic and thereby blocking the deep sharing of experiences that creates true community.

While struggling with historical definitions of power is vital, simple deconstruction is unable to answer adequately the question of how, in this generation, we are to perform power. Third wave feminists must struggle with completely new definitions of power, ones which divorce power from the economic model and, therefore, from its patriarchal roots. We propose relational power as such a conceptualization of power. Relational power, as put forth by Bernard Loomer (1976), rests on a frequently overlooked definition of power: "the capacity for being acted upon or undergoing an effect" (*Merriam-Webster's Dictionary*, 1999). This definition, combined with the understanding that either/or thinking does not beget new knowledge, yields a definition of power as "the ability both to produce and undergo an effect . . . the capacity both to influence others and to be influenced by others" (Loomer, 1976, p. 17). It is important to note there is no "or" in this conception of power; to construe power as the ability to produce *or* undergo an effect would immediately lead to active and passive dichotomies and straight on into the realm of hierarchical power, unilateral influence, and ideological rape. Instead, relational power is the dynamic interplay between two *active* processes in which the ability to be influenced is an active openness to, and inclusion of, another in our world of meaning and concern. This openness, in turn, contains the potential to influence the one to whom we have opened ourselves, who by their own active openness and inclusion may once again influence us.

The language of relational power can seem as convoluted as a Gordian knot rather than the intricately woven Celtic knot actually represented. The difficulty in discussing relational power lies in its radical break from patriarchal, economic, and Western modes of thinking about power, relationship, and the very nature of existence. The English language, so steeped in these traditional systems, has difficulty conveying the dynamism, synergism, mutuality, and interpenetration of relational power. Embedded in these traditional systems of thought is the understanding of power as externally focused and as an economy of exchange, of relationship as fundamentally threatening to individuality, and of human existence as constituted in a bounded, privatized, overdetermined self. By contrast, embedded in the relational system of thought is the understanding of power as the awareness of "the presence of others in our own being" and the ability to sustain this internal mutuality (Loomer, 1976, p. 20), of relationships as the matrix of profound connection in which uniqueness and community flourish (Johnson, 1992), and of human existence as emergent within and inseparable from relationships (Loomer, 1976; Surrey, 1991). There is no economy of exchange or hierarchy in the relational view of power because the principle of equality is not one of *quid pro quo* or magnanimously offering to share power equally, but a realization that "we are equally dependent on the constitutive relationships that create us, however relatively unequal we are in our various strengths . . ." (Loomer, 1976, p. 22). Societal privilege does not determine relational power. Relational power is determined by the degree to which one can actively open to the influence of others' experiences, without losing one's identity or creative freedom. Therefore, relational power is also the ability to hold contrasting experiences in relationship (Loomer, 1976). From this perspective, the greater the contrast held, the greater the relational power. While traditional models of power search for agreement or consensus, this alternate model holds diversity and foundational equality in relationship with one another. Consensus, even radical influencing of others, may happen via relational power; however, such change is never brought about by demonstrations of force and traditional power. Rather, change comes about through the invitation for everyone to focus on the "relationship to which all contribute and from which all members are fed" (Loomer, 1976, pp. 22-23). We believe the third wave of feminism, swelling from the strength of relational power as thus defined, contains the potential to transform the shores of our profession and humanity.

THE THIRD WAVE BREAKING ON THE SHORE

Relational power, in its subversion of dominant conceptualizations and ways of being, creates the possibility for new ways of being. Multiple implications for feminist psychology stem from relational performance of power, and it is to this discussion we now turn.

Broadening and Deepening the Wave

Relational praxis, as defined in this paper, offers a means to deeper dialogue, connection, and community within diversity as feminist psychology continues struggling to reconcile its historical identification as a White, middle-class, educated movement with its desire to value diverse women's experience. Subversion of socially-derived privilege as the coin of power means the narratives of multiply oppressed women no longer need be perceived as threatening to the feminist movement's idea of itself as equality-based. Instead, rooted in a context of simultaneous active opening to and movement towards another, "unity and differentiation [become] correlates rather than opposites of each other" (Johnson, 1992, p. 217) and dialogues between women with diverse experiences, values, and perspectives contain the potential for deep, dynamic mutuality.

Attempting to perform power relationally is difficult because the patriarchy has inculcated us to construe and practice power non-relationally. Therefore, we can easily fall into external forms of relatedness, believing the myth of separate selves and not risking true inclusion of others within ourselves. Relationally powerful dialogue focuses not on the external relationship but on the internal experience of relatedness wherein giving and receiving can "seem to be almost indistinguishable . . . [and] the greatest influence that one can exercise on another consists in being influenced by the other, in enabling the other to make the largest impact on one's self" (Loomer, 1976, p. 22). Entering a dialogue intentionally rooted in relational power involves risk on many levels. At its best, relational power involves the risk of making room for another's suffering–unrationalized and from which one may not distance–within one's self, opening dearly held beliefs and certainties to the possibility of change, and the potential pain associated with growth. At its most dangerous, relational power involves the risk that one person may meet the performance of relational power by another with an exercise of unilateral force. This is especially true when differentials in traditionally defined power exist within relationships, as those high in societal power often feel weakest in relational power, and, threatened, are more likely to respond with a show of force. Relational power as a way of life requires considerably more commitment, energy, active patience, and emotional and psychic strength than traditional modes of power, including egalitarianism. With respect to relationship within diversity, we believe strivings toward relational power are vital to the creation of "genuine mutuality in which there is radical equality while distinctions are respected" (Johnson, 1992, p. 216).

Drawing Strength from the Second Wave

In the earlier sections of this article, we discussed the failure of our generation to integrate the subversive narratives of women's histories into our collective memory. Increases in social power and privilege can provide this generation with access to the social structures that are traditional means of effecting change. However, the higher one is in the traditional power hierarchy, the less awareness of subversive narratives there is and the stronger the temptation for complacency and comfort grows. To take our place fully within feminist psychology, we need to develop equally the sense of ourselves as intimately part of the life-giving waters of previous waves and of our own uniqueness as the third wave.

Mentoring by second wave feminists is one particularly potent antidote to this near amnesia for subversive narratives and sense of disconnection from our history. The third wave needs, again, to hear and attach meaning to the stories of our feminist foremothers. Such mentoring is difficult within the frame of traditional power relationships. Traditional hierarchical power, obviously, blocks true mentoring. Mentoring in this context increases another's power while bringing about the feared concomitant loss of one's own power. On the surface, egalitarianism appears the perfect context for mentoring. However, the unacknowledged hierarchy implicit in this approach to power has consequences for both second and third wave women. As young feminists, we recognize the power differentials resulting from differences in age, experience, and, often, education and class as well. Such differences in traditional power can create passivity on the part of those being mentored, turning mentoring into another academic learning of feminism rather than a true engagement with and integration of our history. In turn, this passive stance can frustrate second wave mentors who are confused as to why their movements toward egalitarianism often do not have the desired effects. At the same time, the attempted repudiation of traditional modes of power through egalitarianism can lead second wave feminists to deny their own importance in the history of feminism and for the development of young feminists. There is a sense that many to whom the third wave would look for mentoring, when faced with this possibility, look around and utter, "Who me? A feminist foremother? You must be mistaken. . . . " We believe the previous generation's discomfort with power leads to this questioning and impedes the mentoring process.

A shift to relational power has profound implications for the mentoring process and the development of young feminists' memory of subversive narratives and our subversive history. Perhaps most importantly, relational power creates a context for active participation by both people in the mentoring relationship. By removing the covert hierarchy and unidirectionality of egalitarianism and focusing on the process of creating mutually internal relationship, relational power makes the passivity of young feminists impossible and reduces the impediments to second wave feminists viewing themselves as foremothers. As with dialogues in diversity, relational power provides for the acknowledgment and discussion of power differentials via the sharing and incorporation of each other's experience so vital to personal and professional development. Further, relational power is, we assert, the only means through which the third wave can come to view itself as indivisible from the ocean of feminism. The restoration of connection is brought about through the relational mentoring process during which young feminists make room for the lives of our fore mothers within our concerns, our personal meanings, and our selves. At the same time, we need both the influence of second wave feminists and their active opening to our influence. In this way, we not only reclaim subversive narratives from previous generations, we also share our own sense of subversion and, in so doing, discover the ontological nature of our connectedness and common history. In this pool of connected unity and diversity, young feminists grow in relational power and praxis, learn the intricacies of feminist psychology, and both generations become more than they could be alone.

Invitation to Swim in the Waters of the Third Wave

As we take our place in the psychological profession, third wave feminists must invite others, clients and colleagues, to come and swim in these new waters. Our invitation, however, must come relationally. Within relational power, we may not require clients or colleagues to become like us in order to receive full inclusion and consideration. Instead, we must engage our professional relationships as a dance of mutual connection in which we may move toward and away and around and within each other's experience, opening ourselves to mutual influencing. Engaging others within the context of relational power is especially important when the "other," whether client or colleague, potentially is viewed as someone who will not "get with the feminist program." Traditional conversations between those with differing perspectives do not contain the potential for change, as each party is trying to get the other to change while remaining unchanged themselves. The performance of relational power facilitates true dialogue and communication while containing no room for escalating power plays. Even if one person in the dialogue chooses to exercise unilateral power, the other still may respond relationally, creating space within themselves and the relationship to be influenced by this show of unilateral power and sharing the experience of being influenced. This very act of opening rather than armoring, while painful, creates the potential for transformation and movement towards mutual relational engagement. Such opening is especially important in the context of therapy, where traditional power differentials exist and armoring and retaliation on the part of the therapist, no matter how well rationalized as "therapeutic," leads to significant client harm (Bruns, 2000). The work of the Stone Center provides an articulate theory for working relationally, whether with clients or colleagues (see, for example, Miller & Stiver, 1997; Fletcher, 1999). Authenticity, zest, and empathy, as well as the ability to maintain connection while disconnected, all arise out of the dynamic waters of relational power. Our hope is that the reconceptualization of power away from egalitarianism toward relational power will create, for all the reasons discussed in this article, a more inviting and more dynamic place for all humanity to swim.

Relational Power: Subverting the Undertow

The performance of relational power within diversity dialogues, mentoring relationships, and our invitations to others to enter the waters of feminism is in its very construction a subversion of the backlash. The myth of separation and the denial of our essential constitution within relationships give strength to the undertow striving to pull society away from radical equality. Our inability truly to communicate with one another in active opening and to maintain mutually internal relationships renders us ineffective swimmers and concerned only for our own well-being when we dive into the waters of patriarchy. The economic model of power, whether hierarchical or egalitarian, fuels the backlash because any movement toward equality is viewed as a loss of power by someone. Loss, in traditional understandings, then engenders a battle to reclaim what was lost while others attempt to preserve what was won.

Relational power is the counterpoint for all that creates and feeds the backlash. In the rising light of relational power, the myth of separation yields to the truth of our fundamental connection and creation within relationship. We must actively open ourselves to all people's experiences, holding simultaneously the commonality and diversity of oppression and suffering. In mutually internal relationships, no one's well-being can stand outside of the third wave's concern. Political activism can be the only result from experiences of such relationality. Relational activism, then, becomes not a kindly response to someone of lesser power's suffering but, rather, the only authentic response to being truly affected by another. Our recognition of our feminist foremothers' subversive narratives as integral to our own identities connects us to the influential power of our heritage. Our movement toward our own performance of power provides new ways of influencing and a means of subverting the patriarchy without relying on the master's tools. And finally, our rhythmic breaking over the shore of humanity, feminist and patriarchal, if the third wave can live into this relational power, holds the potential to transform the face of the beach, creating a place where we can all have value in one another's lives.

REFERENCES

Alfonso, Rita, & Trigilio, Jo (1997). Surfing the third wave: A dialogue between two third wave feminists. *Hypatia* [On-line], 12 (3). Available: http://www.is.csupomona. edu/%7Eljshrage/hypatia/surfing.htm

Alliaume, Karen T., (1998). New feminist theologies: The third wave. *Cross Currents* [On-line], 38. Available: http://www.aril.org/editorial%20summer%201998.htm

American Heritage Dictionary, The (2nd ed.). (1983). New York: Dell Books.

Broverman, Inge K., Broverman, Donald M., Clarkson, Frank E., Rosenkrantz, Paul S., & Vogel, Susan R. (1970). Sex role stereotypes and clinical judgments of mental health. *Journal of Consulting and Clinical Psychology, 34,* 1-7.

Brown, Laura (1994). *Subversive dialogues: Theory in feminist therapy.* New York: Basic Books.

Bruns, Cindy M. (2000). A rose by any other name? Borderline Personality Disorder and Complex PTSD. In C. M. Bruns and P. Birrell (Co-chairs), *Difficult Dialogues: What's in a Word?* Symposium presented at the annual meeting of the Association of Women in Psychology, Salt Lake City, Utah, U.S.A, March 2000.

Chesler, Phyllis (1972). *Women and madness.* New York: Harcourt Brace Jovanovich.

Feminist Therapy Institute (1990). Feminist therapy institute code of ethics. In H. Lerman, & N. Porter (Eds.), *Feminist ethics in psychotherapy* (pp. 37-40). New York: Springer Publishing Company.

Fletcher, Joyce K. (1999). *Disappearing acts: Gender, power, and relational practice at work.* Cambridge, MA: MIT Press.

Friedan, Betty (1963). *The feminine mystique.* New York: Norton.

Gilligan, Carol (1982). *In a different voice: Psychological theory and women's development.* Cambridge, MA: Harvard University Press.

Johnson, Elizabeth A. (1992). *She who is: The mystery of God in feminist theological discourse.* New York: Crossroad Publishing Company.

Jordan, Judith V. (1997). *Women's growth in diversity.* New York: Guilford Press.

Josefowitz Siegel, Rachel, & Larsen, Carolyn (1990). The ethics of power differentials. In H. Lerman, & N. Porter (Eds.), *Feminist ethics in psychotherapy* (pp. 41-42). New York: Springer Publishing Company.

Kanuha, Valli (1990). The need for an integrated analysis of oppression in feminist therapy ethics. In H. Lerman, & N. Porter (Eds.), *Feminist ethics in psychotherapy* (pp. 24-35). New York: Springer Publishing Company.

Lerman, Hannah, & Rigby, Dorothe N. (1990). Boundary violations: Misuse of the power of the therapist. In H. Lerman, & N. Porter (Eds.), *Feminist ethics in psychotherapy* (pp. 51-59). New York: Springer Publishing Company.

Loomer, Bernard (1976). Two conceptions of power. *Process Studies, 6 (1),* 5-32.

Merriam-Webster's Collegiate Dictionary (10th ed.). (1999). Springfield, MA: Merriam-Webster, Inc.

Miller, Jean B. (1976). *Toward a new psychology of women (2nd ed.).* Boston, MA: Beacon Press.

Miller, Jean B. (1987). Women and power. *Women & Therapy, 6 (1/2),* 1-10.

Miller, Jean B., & Stiver, Irene P. (1997). *The healing connection.* Boston, MA: Beacon Press.

Surrey, J. L. (1991). The "self-in-relation": A theory of women's development. In J. V. Jordan, A. G. Kaplan, J. B. Miller, J. P. Stiver and J. L. Surrey (Eds.), *Women's growth in connection* (pp. 51-66) NY: Guilford.

The Trouble with Power

Cindy B. Veldhuis

SUMMARY. Power in therapy is an issue of great import. As feminist therapists, we work to create a relationship in which power is shared, and where mutuality is the goal. Yet denying power differentials in the therapy relationship may have deleterious consequences. Believing that we are powerless or have no power relative to others may be one of the most important issues related to harm in therapy. This article explores the ways in which a lack of recognition of power may be damaging through a discussion of women's relationship to power, power in therapy, and how denial of power may be associated with harm in therapy relationships. *[Article copies available for a fee from The Haworth Document Delivery Service: 1-800-342-9678. E-mail address: <getinfo@haworthpressinc.com> Website: <http://www.HaworthPress.com> © 2001 by The Haworth Press, Inc. All rights reserved.]*

KEYWORDS. Power, therapy, feminist therapy, powerlessness, mutuality, abuse of power, boundary violations, therapist-client relationships

Cindy B. Veldhuis is affiliated with the Psychology Department, University of Illinois, Chicago, IL. Address correspondence to: Cindy Veldhuis, Department of Psychology, 1007 W. Harrison, m/c 285, University of Illinois at Chicago, Chicago, IL 60607 (E-mail: cveldh1@uic.edu).

The author gratefully acknowledges the support and assistance of Pam Birrell, Tracy Caldwell, Angela Miller, Len Newman, Stephanie Riger, Linda Skitka, and Catherine Sloat-Leiper. She would like especially to thank Liz Dooley and Jennifer Freyd, without whom this could not have been written.

[Haworth co-indexing entry note]: "The Trouble with Power." Veldhuis, Cindy B. Co-published simultaneously in *Women & Therapy* (The Haworth Press, Inc.) Vol. 23, No. 2, 2001, pp. 37-56; and: *The Next Generation: Third Wave Feminist Psychotherapy* (ed: Ellyn Kaschak) The Haworth Press, Inc., 2001, pp. 37-56. Single or multiple copies of this article are available for a fee from The Haworth Document Delivery Service [1-800-342-9678, 9:00 a.m. - 5:00 p.m. (EST). E-mail address: getinfo@haworthpressinc.com].

in the wind/lost breaths wishes
dying for someone to loom over the horizon
anyone/come talk/please come talk to me/now
before I forget how & become silence.

–Ntozake Shange, 1987

INTRODUCTION

As therapists, we seek to "hear another to speech" (Heyward, 1993) and to end silence about such issues as violence, oppression, hate, and inequality. Feminist psychology additionally has, at its core, the tenet that as psychologists we must aim not only to help the individual, but also to shape society in such a way that distress of the individual is lessened. Further, the Feminist Therapy Institute's Ethical Code states that it is an ethical imperative that feminist therapists "end inequities . . . through cultural transformation and radical social change" (Brown, 1994, p. 19), and that this needs to be a goal of therapy as well. Part of how we attempt to meet these goals is by redefining power, analyzing its impact on our clients' lives, and working to give the client power (Wyche & Rice, 1997). In helping the client feel her own power in the therapy relationship, she may perhaps experience power in other parts of her life (Marecek & Kravetz, 1998).

Power in therapy is an issue of great import. Not only do we work to help the client find her own power, we also work to decrease the power differential found in traditional therapy relationships (Douglas & Walker, 1988). Through this more egalitarian relationship, the client will hopefully find herself in a safe and trusting relationship through which she can locate her voice, her truths, and effect change in her life.

WOMEN AND POWER

A friend once likened power to the flame of a candle. When the flame of the lit candle is shared with those who need their own candles lit, it does not diminish the flame; rather, it adds to the surrounding warmth and light. When power is shared, it does not deplete; instead, it gives others power, and that can only enhance. Nevertheless, many people believe that power is a finite resource. If one person has power, then others do not.

In a culture where power is seen as a limited resource, many, especially women, believe that they have no power (Lips, 1994). Because women are societally in a place of lesser power, and attempts to gain some modicum of power are thwarted regularly, it may be difficult to understand how one may have any power whatsoever. In the therapy role, however, it may in fact be deleterious not to recognize one's own power (Brown, 1994). Believing that we are powerless or have no power relative to others is likely one of the most important issues related to harm in therapy (Lerman & Rigby, 1990).

Early feminist therapy sought to level the power playing field. In order to redress the power imbalances and abuses in traditional therapy, feminist therapists wanted to create a therapeutic relationship in which power was equal. However, as Laura Brown (1994) states, early feminist therapy was created in rebellion against traditional therapy, and as such, may not always be in line with what the client needs; rather it is in reaction to what we think the client does not need. We know that clients do not need a "blank screen" therapist; nor do they need a therapist who is the expert on the client's life, nor a therapist with rigid boundaries who insists on being called Doctor. Conversely, clients also do not need a friend in their therapist, a date, nor a therapist with no boundaries. Somewhere between the two poles exists the paradigm for feminist therapy, and perhaps finding this paradigm is a task young feminists can tackle.

Equal power is neither possible nor perhaps in line with therapeutic goals. Although well-intentioned, early attempts to equalize power led some therapists to see clients as peers who did not need special protections from boundary transgressions (Brown, 1994). Rather than completely obliterating power imbalances, it perhaps behooves therapists instead to be aware of the power imbalance, to use power consciously and wisely, and to assist the client in creating her own ways of having comparable amounts of power. Moreover, it is not enough simply to be aware that a power imbalance exists. The therapist must also work to understand how the power imbalance may affect the client, and further the therapist must be keenly aware of her position as the one with the power.

This article seeks to understand the ways in which a lack of recognition of power may be harmful. In building on some of the formative theorizing and clinical experiences of Laura Brown and Hannah Lerman, I examine why this lack of recognition of power is problematic, and I theorize about the process through which feeling powerless becomes problematic. In doing so, my hope is that we can find ways to avoid this in our own clinical work, and to recognize warning signs in our colleagues. In order to examine how this denial of power may be problematic, I draw upon various psychological literatures and sources: social, community, developmental, clinical psychologies, feminist therapy, feminist psychology, and when possible, writings about clients' experiences, as well as my own clinical experiences.

Women's Paradoxical Relationship with Power

Power is ubiquitous, yet difficult to define (Yoder & Kahn, 1992). Foucault defines power as the manner in which people "are given a location and subjectivity as actors within discourse" (Sampson, p. 1223). To have power is to have the energy, ability, or agency to control, to act, to affect, to do, to produce, to impact, or to influence oneself, others, events, or feelings.

Power is dynamic and may be temporal. It can change based on the context, the relationship or the time (Unger, 1986); that is, someone may have power in one context or time period, but none in another. Griscom (1992) states that a definition of power must, therefore, be one that does not involve just coercion or dominance. It must be defined as relational, it must be contextual, and it must be dynamic.

Power may in fact have both negative and positive connotations for women. It may at once be seen as something corrupt, dangerous, and imbued with oppressive innuendoes (Kitzinger, 1992). Paradoxically, it is something to be attained, something that elevates, foments revolution, is creative and opens up opportunities. In a 1992 study, Miller and Cummins found that 74% women tend to think of societally defined power as "control over." When asked how they defined power for themselves, they defined it as "personal authority" (86.8%). As Kitzinger (1992) states, it seems as though there are two different conceptions of power, male power or power-over (which is "bad" and is typically associated with dominance, control, and coercion) and female power or power-with (which is "good," and is associated with empowerment, shared power, and connection).

Although seeing power as having two forms–power-over vs. power-with–has assisted the field in finding non-coercive ways of having power, it has also created a dichotomous category, which tends to imply connotations of good and bad. Feminist writers have long been aware that dichotomies are artificial. Any time there is a dichotomous category, one will always inherently be seen as superior, and the other as inferior (Sampson, 1993). It is difficult to think of any contradictions, e.g., thin/fat, rich/poor, white/black, straight/gay, man/woman, sane/crazy.

Why is this? According to Gatens (1991), when there are two categories A and B, a whole continuum of possibilities becomes lumped into either A or B. Further, A is by definition positive, encompassing all that is good in the continuum, and thus B becomes Not-A. That is, B is then seen as A's opposite, and is composed of all that is not captured in A, "Not-A becomes the privation or absence of A; the fact that it is Not-A is what defines it, rather than the fact that it is B" (p. 93). For example, if we apply this to gender, we see that man is A, and woman is therefore Not-A. "Woman is an incomplete man" (Sampson, 1993, p. 1224) because man is the cultural ideal, and woman is, therefore, held up and defined against man.

Following this argument, if, as feminists, we see power-to as A—that is, power-to as the ideal and the implicit standard for how power ought be used, then power-over becomes Not-A. We might then associate all situations in which we inherently have power over another negatively. If the definition of power held in one's head is the "bad" or masculine one, then one will likely have an idea of power equating dominance, power over, abuse, and control. This is not the kind of power for which feminist therapists typically strive. "Few feminist therapists seem willing to be caught in the act of being powerful" (Brown, 1994, p. 106).

Why might one feel she is powerless when in a role of power? Women in American society have less structural, social and interpersonal power than do men (Lips, 1994). This may have an impact on women's perceptions of their own power, and cause them to be unaware in certain situations (such as in a therapy relationship) that they possess power. They may therefore see their relationships with clients as equal when they are in fact unequal. Because women have less structural, social, and interpersonal power, they may be motivated not to engage in unequal power relationships.

Women may also not be given much motivation to embrace power. Women who appear powerful, confident, and competent are more likely to be rejected than either men with these traits, or women who are self-effacing and passive (Carli, 1999). This is further complicated by the issue of the one area in which women have increased power over men—referent power. Referent power is power through perceived likeability or social attractiveness (Carli, 1999). Ironically, if a woman asserts her competence and confidence in order to gain power, she may actually end up being ill-perceived, and then is at risk for losing referent power. Power may further have a negative connotation, and as a result, women therapists may feel uncomfortable in positions of increased power, resulting perhaps in denial of having increased power over another. In a qualitative study with 25 therapists, Marecek and Kravetz (1998) investigated their feelings about feminist therapy. In particular, the therapists identified power as a troubling issue, and even had difficulty using the word power in reference to therapy (Marecek & Kravetz, 1998). In discussing power, they used the language of empowerment versus oppression, good versus bad power, masculine versus feminine power, and internal versus external power. Power seems very dichotomized to these feminist therapists, and there seems to be a clear sense of power that is to be espoused and power to be eschewed.

Feminist therapists may in fact choose to deny any power rather than be associated with negative power. Yet even power-over may be useful (Griscom, 1992). Parents' power over their children can be used to create safety or to create boundaries for the child to assist in their development. As will be discussed in the next section, power-over can be useful even in a therapy relationship.

WHAT IS POWER IN THERAPY?

Brown (1994) discusses two definitions of power within therapy relationships: structural and symbolic. Structural power is the power the therapist has resultant from her role in the therapy relationship. The therapist has power to charge fees, set times, end sessions, end therapy, determine diagnoses, choose the setting for therapy, etc. Symbolic power relates to the power of the context of the therapy relationship for the client and the meaning the therapist has in the client's life. Although the client, in effect, hires the therapist to provide a service, giving her some power, the client comes to the therapist, typically, in need, in a vulnerable time in her life. Given her emotional vulnerability, the client may, at the outset, see herself as the one with lesser power.

The therapist's use of power can either harm or assist the client in her therapeutic process. Structural power creates a unique relationship that is different from friendships, familial or intimate relationships. This power sets the relationship apart, makes it distinct and has the potential to create a safe place where the client knows what the rules are, and what the limits are. This power further allows her to explore things in a way that is deeper than would be afforded by a relationship without this structural power differential. Mutuality and empowerment are to be found within this power differential, not through eradication of it (Eldridge, Mencher & Slater, 1997).

Problems with Mutuality

Attempts to equalize the power in therapy may in fact be counterproductive and may create a false sense of equality. In a discussion of empowerment within the domain of community psychology, Riger (1993) states that when attempts to empower individuals are made through increased participation or changes in procedures, the individuals may feel more empowered. However Riger states, "empowerment is sometimes equated with participation, as if changing procedures will automatically lead to changes in the context or distribution of resources" (p. 282). Although empowered individuals may perceive an increase in control, their actual power may be negligible.

How does this relate to a therapy relationship? If the therapist sets out to create an equal and mutual relationship, and desires to empower her clients to have equal power, she may only achieve a false sense of equality. The context of the therapy relationship is unchanged. Therapy relationships are inherently unequal: a client comes in with needs, the therapist assists. The client discloses and becomes more vulnerable, and while the therapist may disclose and also become vulnerable, because of her position in the relationship she is still the one with power. The therapist collects a fee, decides (ultimately) when and where therapy will occur, when therapy ends, and if the therapist ends therapy, this has very different meaning than if the client ends therapy.

Despite a therapist's attempts at mutuality and assisting the client in becoming an expert of her own life, the therapist is often seen as the expert. Yet feminist therapists have long grappled with the uncomfortable idea of therapist as expert (Brown, 1994). There has been great emphasis on helping the client to see herself as the expert on her own life. Feminist therapists also work to depathologize distress, and to assist clients to see the symptoms of distress as normal reactions to abnormal circumstances (Brown, 1994).

Yet in doing so, we may forget the power that comes with our degrees and the letters after our names. Psychologists are instilled by the public with great cognitive authority (Addelson, 1993). When a psychologist says something, whether it is in the consulting room, on a talk show, in the newspaper, or even at a social occasion, it is likely that, as a function of our training and degrees, what we say will be given great credence.

In a survey of women and their therapists, Lott (1999) found that over 75% (N = 274) indicated feelings of love or attachment for their therapists. The therapist becomes larger than life and holds great relational power and meaning in the client's life.

> Women enter therapy with great hopes and high anxiety. They long for comfort and support, insight and understanding, to feel better and to make fundamental changes in their lives. They suspend disbelief and put their trust in the therapist's presumably superior knowledge. They assume that the therapist will be able to see things themselves that they cannot see, will help them to change what seems intractable. (Lott, 1999, p. 65-66)

Because of this set of expectations, the therapist is seen as someone with a great deal of power, even if the therapist works hard to break down the power imbalances or does not see herself as having great power. This is typically the only therapy relationship for the client, but the client is just one of many for the therapist (Eldridge, Mencher & Slater, 1997). The relationship has great power for the client. The client is also likely to keep the therapist with her even when she is not in therapy as, "the half-life of transference [exceeds] that of plutonium" (Hall, 1984 as cited by Eldridge, Mencher & Slater, 1997). Clients may think about their therapist outside of the therapy hour, write to them in their journals, imagine conversations between the two of them, and hold the therapist in their head, as an internalized commentator on their life (Brown, 1994). When we think about our power in these terms, it is a bit humbling, to say the least.

POWERLESSNESS AS PARADOX

Defensive projection might shed some more light on why feeling powerless may be harmful in therapy. Defensive projection means simply that if someone has an unwanted trait, they may see it magnified in others (Newman, Duff, & Baumeister, 1997). If one is motivated not to have power, she may dislike the part of herself that has power. For example, if a therapist feels uncomfortable being in a position of power, she may then dislike that aspect of herself. There may be, in the therapy relationship, constant reminders of the therapist's power. She must therefore work to inhibit awareness of this discrepancy in order to maintain a schema of equivalent power (Newman et al., 1997).

Despite the inhibition of awareness of power over another, "what is left repressed, or what cannot be uttered, is often as significant to the whole shape of the life as what is said" (Braham, 1995, p. 37 as cited by Fivush, 1997). Repressed thoughts or feelings still have an impact. They may shape behavior, cause psychological distress, or somatic symptomology. In order not to think about or feel something, the information must be inhibited, and the more upsetting the thought or feeling, the more energy it takes to inhibit (Pennebaker, 1997). Unresolved material is likely to leak out in some form. The more one works to inhibit, the more it becomes chronically accessible (Newman et al., 1997). If a therapist works hard to deny power, that power then becomes increasingly chronically accessible as the therapist actively tries to deny it. According to the theory of defensive projection, this may then cause the attribution of the disliked part of the self onto another. In the process, this negative schema perhaps then becomes projected upon the client. As a result, if a therapist has high structural power, but dislikes that, she may deny her power, and incorrectly project increased power onto another.

Put simply, if I have power in a therapy relationship, but I really really do not want that power, I will work hard to suppress knowledge that I possess that power. Then, because I am working so hard to suppress my thoughts of my own power, there is a rebound effect (Newman et al., 1997) such that that power becomes the lens through which I see everything. I then see power in everyone around me, and I see myself as not having power. I am perhaps then at risk for seeing my clients as having increased power over me, and myself as powerless.

That Power Becomes You

Denied power is power run amok (Brown, 1994). If a therapist sees herself as powerless, then perhaps by default, she is likely to see the other as the one with power. Women, according to Miller and Cummins (1992), are most likely to feel powerless when they feel a lack of personal control or feel the other person has more power than they do. Low perceived power therapists may attribute increased power to a client, who actually has very little power in the relationship. When in a position of lower perceived power, college students tended to use "bad" interpersonal power strategies, such as telling, laissez-faire, bargaining, negative affect and withdrawal, more often than when they felt they had equivalent or increased power (Sagrestano, 1992).

Bugental et al. (1999) state that feeling as though one has no power, when the person is actually in a position of power, may cause her to defend against the other person, and ironically to view the other as the one with the power. In their studies of parents, Bugental and her colleagues have found that low-power parents demonstrate increased levels of negative affect when their children are unresponsive or respond in ways that upset the parent. The parent further works to regain control of the child. The parents may then be prone to using coercion in order to get what they need and to increase their own sense of power and self-worth (Bugental et al., 1999). If the therapist feels that she is in a place of decreased power, and in the moment incorrectly believes that the client has the upper hand, Bugental and her colleagues' findings would suggest that the therapist is likely to respond in a way that reasserts power, and in effect, harms the client.

Coercive tactics are further associated with therapist burnout (McCarthy & Frieze, 1999). In a study of college students who had been in therapy, participants were asked to rate their therapists' perceived levels of burnout and power tactics. Therapists who were rated as exhibiting signs of burnout (emotional exhaustion, depersonalization, and reduced personal accomplishment) were more likely to use coercive tactics (i.e., therapist is sarcastic, avoids eye contact, does not listen or becomes frustrated) in therapy. Burnout and coercive tactics are also associated with decreases in client satisfaction and with termination resultant from dissatisfaction with therapy. There has been little research on powerlessness and burnout, but it appears that the two are associated (Powell, 1994) such that powerlessness may be a risk factor for burnout.

Perhaps even more troubling is the association between coercive power and others' perceptions. Those who exhibit coercive power are perceived by others as having the power to punish. If a therapist utilizes coercive power, and is perceived by her clients as having the power to punish, this may then introduce fear into the client, which is decidedly countertherapeutic and perhaps extremely harmful. If the client is in fear of the therapist or is feeling coerced by the therapist, she may feel she has no voice, power, or agency within the relationship and is therefore in an exceptionally vulnerable position. Ironically, extreme denial of our own power may cause us to create a dynamic in which our client feels she must comply, and we, without even knowing it, are in a position of dominance. We may be, therefore, playing out the very power differences we wish to avoid.

Feelings of powerlessness may also cause one to dismiss any potential for harm they may have in the relationship and, further, to pathologize or deny any distress the client may express as a result of the harm wrought. At the extreme end, abusers (batterers, sexual perpetrators, and abusive parents) see themselves as victims, the ones without power (Bugental et al., 1999; Veldhuis & Freyd, 1999). Because they believe they are the ones who have been victimized, they place the onus on the actual victim. Freyd (1996) calls this "Deny Attack Reverse Victim-Offender" (as part of her DARVO model of the methods perpetrators use to deny culpability when victims disclose abuse), and has theorized that it is actually a powerful strategy for avoiding responsibility and for making the victim feel that she is the one to blame.

In a therapy relationship in which there have been ethical violations, the use of this strategy might be particularly problematic. If a therapist harms a client, and then reverses the victim-offender status in order to reduce her own culpability, as a result of her position as therapist, she can cause great harm to the client. Because of the cognitive authority of the therapist, because she has access to information about the client's functioning, and intimate details about the client and the issues that bring the client to therapy, it is likely that she will be believed. As will be discussed in the next section, the very fact that the client is a client automatically discredits her should she seek assistance in resolving ethical issues arising from the therapeutic relationship. If the ethically problematic therapist further states that the client is the one who behaved in a problematic manner, whose narrative is likely to be given credence? Moreover, what might this do to the client? If the client feels harmed as a result of ethical issues in therapy, voices these concerns and is told by the therapist that it is in fact her fault, is she in a position to question the therapist's words? I would argue that it is very likely that she would internalize the blame, locate the onus for the ethical problems in herself, and that this could be very harmful to the well-being of the client. This is perhaps the most harmful result of denial of power in a therapy relationship.

Impact of Powerlessness Run Amok

Typologies of boundary violations have their roots in the power differential (Brown, 1994). Peterson (1992) outlines four characteristics of boundary violations: reversal of roles, secrecy, double binds, and the indulgence of personal privilege. It is easy to see how the desire for power, or feeling excess power-over one's client could cause the exploitation or abuse of a client. It is less apparent, however, how the denial of increased power could also lead to abuses.

When a therapist relies on the client to attend to the therapist's own needs, reversal of roles has occurred. This can be a very subtle and seemingly harmless reversal, such as Brown's (1994) example of the therapist who looks forward to a certain client because the client laughs at the therapist's jokes and makes the therapist feel good about herself. This characteristic of a boundary violation can also be seen in the more extreme example of a therapist who asks a client for a hug in order to alleviate her own distress (Lott, 1999). A therapist who denies her place of greater power in the therapeutic relationship will likely see such violations as part of an egalitarian relationship. However, even seemingly innocuous boundary violations may have a great impact on the client. The client may feel concurrently pleased at the attention, yet confused by it: "Clients mistakenly believe that feeling special stems from who they are as people. . . . In reality they are only special because of their ability to minister to the professional's needs" (Peterson, 1992, p. 78).

As a result, the client is unaware of the therapist's actual intent. Is the special attention part of the therapeutic intent? Or is it solely to meet the needs of the therapist? Is there some ulterior motive? Because the client does not have all the information she needs in order to accurately assess the situation, she may become confused and doubt her reality. An example in Peterson's book is that of a woman who sought assistance from her minister. In their sessions, he had her read from her journal to him, and encouraged her to talk about her sexual feelings. She felt pleased to be able to talk openly about her sexuality, yet also felt uncomfortable. When she expressed her discomfort she was chided for being "uptight." The woman stated, "I would feel there must be something wrong with me that I couldn't talk about it. . . . Instead of feeling good about myself, I felt more ashamed" (p. 84). The hidden agenda (the minister's own arousal) caused her to doubt her reality and to do things that were uncomfortable for her. Had she known of his intent, what were her choices? To confront him, and thus risk losing the connection she had with him? To continue with him would have put her at further risk of exploitation. This dilemma is caused when the options available to the client put her in an impossible position; to continue an ethically problematic relationship, or to end it and lose a perhaps vital connection.

In another example, a client who was a professional writer was asked by his therapist to collaborate on a book with her (Peterson, 1992). Because the therapist did not recognize the impact her position of power had on his ability to consent freely or not to her request, she placed him in a difficult spot. The client stated, "At first I felt flattered.

When I later realized she was using me, I felt furious. I would like to have told her how angry I was, but I couldn't. I still needed the group and didn't want to make her mad" (p. 86).

Clients may also resist seeing the truth, as to recognize the betrayal means that the person with whom she has likely formed a strong connection is causing her harm. As a result, she may blame herself rather than the therapist and locate the source of the boundary violations in the self. In doing so, she can remain blind to the betrayals, and continue the necessary attachment to her therapist (Freyd, 1997). To speak of the betrayals causes her not only to risk losing her relationship with the therapist, but also to risk being pathologized by those outside of the relationship. She may further fear risking the therapist's reputation or even career. Silence and self-blame may thus be the safest options.

Expecting that a client can be fully involved in a discussion of ethical dilemmas is still problematic, although on the right track. It should of course be the goal that the client have a voice, but it is also of extreme importance to realize that the client may not feel fully free to engage in such a discussion for fear of upsetting or losing the therapist. Further, clients may not have a full understanding of the range of issues at stake. For example, if a therapist is discussing potential dual relational issues with a client (e.g., becoming friends after termination), the client may feel pleased at the idea of having that type of relationship with the therapist. However, the client likely does not have all the information she needs to make that sort of decision, or fully understand the ramifications of such a relationship. She may place at the forefront the therapist's needs, in order to please her or to avoid the risk of losing the therapist's approval. This becomes an issue of informed consent. We need to make clients a part of these difficult discussions, but we must also make certain that they are informed enough to either consent or not, and we must be aware that because of the inherent power differentials, they may not feel completely free to consent or dissent.

Clients may also downplay their feelings or experiences in the face of our degrees. Our cognitive authority and societal position may cause the client to believe that we know what is best, and defer to us: "I didn't think that what he did was inappropriate because I saw him as a counselor with credentials after his name" (Peterson, 1992, p. 86). If we understand that by the very virtue of our profession, we may cause a client to disregard her own intuitions, we can use that awareness to assist them in listening to themselves. However, if we deny this power, we risk causing our clients to deny their own voices.

These issues are highlighted in a compelling example of a therapist who initiated a friendship with her client (Lott, 1999). The client stated that when her therapist spoke kindly to her it had "a greater impact than a thousand compliments from anyone else" (p. 113), and that it was the first time she had ever felt understood or cared for. Thus, the therapist had great symbolic power in the client's life. When the therapist began disclosing aspects of herself to the client so that they could "just be two human beings together" (p. 113), the client felt special. Further, the suggestion to do things outside of therapy felt like "a dream come true" (p. 113), as the therapy relationship had been a particularly powerful and trusting one. Problems erupted, however, causing the client to feel in a double bind. To speak meant risking both the therapy relationship and the friendship. Lott (1999) further notes that in this example, the relationship is far more meaningful to the client than to the therapist due to the "symbolic weight of their emblematic, highly charged . . . therapy relationship" (p. 114). In denying her place of power in the client's life, the therapist created a falsely egalitarian relationship, misused the therapy relationship to meet her own needs, and put the client in a bind in which there was no way she could raise concerns or objections without deleterious consequences.

It is also perhaps time to examine how it is that we as a profession deal with problems in therapy. Laura Brown (1990) has suggested guidelines on how to deal with ethically problematic colleagues. When possible, it is best for all concerned to assist the therapist in understanding the issues and in making the therapy relationship a strong one again. What if, however, this is not possible? What if the therapist's transgressions are too great, or if consultation fails, or if the client and therapist never seek outside assistance? When consultation fails or is not sought, the client is then likely to drop out of therapy, to file ethics complaints, or to perhaps stay in therapy at great risk to herself. None of these is a great option, and sadly, when a client files ethical complaints the process may be difficult at best. When clients file complaints, they are discredited for the very reason that they are there: they sought mental health services, which may immediately cause others to discount their concerns (Wendling, 1999). In the process of reviewing an ethical complaint, the client's chart may be entered into evidence, and as a result, issues that had only been shared with the therapist are now a part of the decision-making process, and may be used to discredit the client.

POWER AND ETHICS

The Feminist Therapy Institute's (FTI) Code of Ethics (1999) creates valuable guidelines for the practice of therapy and especially the issues of power in therapy which go beyond questions of legality to morality. These guidelines were not created to keep feminist therapists free from legal tussles in the event a client is harmed or dissatisfied. Instead, the ethical code creates a set of guidelines for moral, ethical, and humane practice. It encompasses not only what is best for the therapist, but also what is best for the client. Further, it does not set up a list of "thou shalt nots" (Brown, 1994; Feminist Therapy Institute, 1999); rather, it entreats and entrusts the therapist to monitor well the therapy relationship and to use her/his own best judgment of what is needed in each situation.

Because training programs do little to prepare therapists for ethical quandries outside of those covered by the APA ethical guidelines (Eldridge, Mencher & Slater, 1997), it is important for therapists to equip themselves with the self- and client-awareness necessary to deal with ambiguous ethical issues. What information do therapists need in order to make sound client-focused decisions in therapy? How do we "monitor such relationships to prevent potential abuse of or harm to the client" (Lerman & Porter, 1990).

A feminist therapist must have the ability to self-monitor and know fully her/his impact on the client, as well as understand the power differential between the therapist and the client, and the ramifications this power difference may have. Further, the therapist must be able to tell if she is behaving in an ethically questionable way, and have the resources to get assistance if she were to determine that the therapy relationship has gone awry. Finally, she must have the personal wherewithal to recognize when she is hurting her client, and the accountability to put the client's needs at the forefront.

CONCLUSIONS

My only advice is to stay aware, listen carefully and yell for help if you need it.

–Judy Blume, 1986

FTI's ethical guidelines provide a strong moral code for feminist therapists, but how do we ensure that we have the requisite knowledge, skills and self-awareness to navigate the ethical dilemmas certain to come our way? Like Judy Blume, I have little to offer in the way of advice on how not to get sucked into the paradox of powerlessness, except to state that we must stay aware of the power we have, we must listen carefully to our clients, encourage open questioning and create an environment in which clients feel free to state the uncomfortable and the verboten, and we must yell for help if we feel that things have run amok (or are even at risk of running slightly amok).

Stay Aware

I think first we must reconceptualize power as a continuum rather than a good/bad dichotomy, and thus not be afraid of our power. In truly embracing a continuum of gender, for example, we have begun to see the variations as all having worth and viability. It then follows that if we can move to see power as a continuum, then perhaps we can have a more positive view of power and all its variations and applications. Gray areas can be fairly scary, ambiguous, and unsettling; however, as in the gender example, the gray has great value for the field and humanity. Perhaps the grays of power can as well.

In accepting all the power variants, we can, without fear, recognize and make explicit and known the power imbalances, and figure out how to make them work, to protect client and self. Power is not inherently good or bad; it is how we wield it or deny it that gives it negative or positive connotations. When we make explicit the structural and symbolic power imbalances in therapy, we validate our clients' experiences. Laura Brown's definition of egalitarian gives credence to the idea of power imbalance as a useful aspect of therapy:

> there is an equality of value and of respect for each person's worth between the participants, but there continues to be some asymmetry in certain aspects of the exchange, in part designed to empower the less powerful person, but primarily required to define and delineate the responsibilities of the more powerful one. (Brown, p. 104)

Therapists who fail to recognize their own place of increased power in the relationship in effect negate a client's reality (Brown, 1994). Clients typically see us as having some structural or symbolic power, and when we deny that, we deny their reality, and are at risk for losing our ability to understand the relationship from their perspective. When we are aware of our power, we are consciously aware of how our actions, or inactions, affect the client. We recognize that even a brief discontinuation of eye contact may signal something profound to the client. Rather than deny and problematize this power, we must make it explicit and use it to benefit our relationships with our clients. If that eye contact flickers, and we see the impact in the client's face, we can use our power to attend to the moment, and discuss what happened. In doing so, we introduce a new power into the relationship, the power of mutual respect (Siegel & Larson, 1990).

Listen Carefully

"I need to apprehend reality not as I would feel it in their shoes but as they feel it" (Hoagland, 1991, p. 249). In listening to our clients, we give them power. When we understand the power we potentially have in our clients' lives, it helps us to better understand their lived experience. Listening may be painful if we do things that cause our client to hurt, but it is necessary for ethical and healthy therapeutic relationships.

Perhaps an arena into which young feminists can take the field is in assisting clients to have a greater voice. There are few client voices on the issues of feminist therapy, power, and boundary violations. Yet, just as we as individual therapists seek to make the work we do be informed by our clients, perhaps so ought the field. Ostensibly, whenever we write about therapy, our writings are informed by our clients' experiences and perhaps even our own experiences as clients in therapy, but the veil of the therapists' voice may mask the authenticity of the clients' words. Because of our power and meaning in their lives, clients may edit their experiences for us in order to please. We may also edit those experiences, or our own, for fear of appearing a "bad therapist." Perhaps then this may mean that more research ought to be done about clients' experiences with feminist therapists, or the utilization of client focus groups, or perhaps even special journal issues with writings by clients.

Additionally, ensuring that clients have a place to go if they feel their rights or needs have been violated in therapy is perhaps a need young feminists can tackle. Currently, the avenues for clients who have concerns about the care they are receiving in therapy are perhaps not set up to provide the best assistance for clients. As mentioned previously, clients who report ethically problematic psychologists are often discounted because of the fact they sought mental health treatment in the first place

(Wendling, 1999). Clients may further feel ashamed for seeking therapy, or may worry about the confidentiality of their mental health issues were they to file a complaint, and may thus be loath to report the therapist. Thus, perhaps as young feminists we can find safer, less stigmatizing venues for clients with concerns about their therapy.

Yell for Help If You Need It

As Lerman and Rigby (1990) state, if you are concerned about power or boundary issues in therapy, "run, do not walk to your nearest ethically informed feminist therapy colleague(s)" (p. 57). We are all likely, at some point in our careers, to deny our power, to misstep a boundary, or to inadvertently hurt a client. It is in our best interest, as well as the client's, to seek consultation. It may also be of use to let clients know with whom they may consult if they feel uncomfortable at any time. In part, we may deny our power because it can be exhausting to have to attend to every nuance and potential hurt. This exhaustion may well be a signal that we are not ensuring that our own needs are being met. Self-care is vital for therapists, and when we are unable to get our own needs met through our personal relationships and outside of the therapy, we are at increased risk of trying to meet them through our clients. In turn, ensuring that our emotional, physical and cognitive needs are met outside of therapy can have a profoundly positive impact on our work and on our clients (Faunce, 1990).

"I must be able to assess my relationship for abuse/oppression and withdraw if I find it to be so. I feel no guilt, I have grown, I have learned something. I understand my part in the relationship. I separate, I will not go there again. Far from diminishing my ethical self, I am enhancing it" (Hoagland, 1991, p. 256). Understanding our power, getting consultation when we need it, making power differentials explicit and a part of good and safe therapy can only assist us in our growth as clinicians, as well as assist in the growth of our clients.

REFERENCES

Addelson, Kathryn Pyne. (1993). Knowers/doers and their moral problems. In L. Alcoff and E. Potter (Eds.), *Feminist Epistemologies* (pp. 265-294). New York: Routledge.

Blume, J. (1986). *Letters to Judy: What your kids wish they could tell you.* G. P. Putnam's Sons Publishers: New York, p. 94.

Brown, L. S. (1990). Confronting Ethically Problematic Behaviors in Feminist Therapist Colleagues. In H. Lerman and N. Porter (Eds.), *Feminist Ethics in Psychotherapy* (pp. 147-159): Springer Publishing Co.

Brown, L. S. (1994). Subversive dialogues: Theory in feminist therapy. New York, NY, USA: Basicbooks, Inc.

Bugental, D. B., & Lewis, J. C. (1998). Interpersonal power repair in response to threats to control from dependent others. In M. Kofta, G. Weary et al. (Eds.), Personal control in action: Cognitive and motivational mechanisms. The Plenum series in social/clinical psychology. (pp. 341-362). New York, NY, USA: Plenum Press.

Bugental, D. B., Lewis, J. C., Lin, E., Lyon, J., & Kopeikin, H. (1999). In charge but not in control: The management of teaching relationships by adults with low perceived power. *Developmental Psychology*, 35 (6), 1367-1378.

Carli, L. L. (1999). Gender, interpersonal power, and social influence. *Journal of Social Issues*, 55 (1), 81-99.

Douglas, M. A. D., & Walker, L. E. A. (1988). Introduction to feminist therapies. In M. A. D. Douglas & L. E. A. Walker (Eds.), Feminist psychotherapies: Integration of therapeutic and feminist systems (pp. 3-11). Norwood, N J: Ablex Publishing Corporation.

Eldridge, N. S., Mencher, J., & Slater, S. (1997). The conundrum of mutuality: A lesbian dialogue. In J. V. Jordan et al. (Eds.), Women's growth in diversity: More writings from the Stone Center. (pp. 107-137). New York, NY, USA: The Guilford Press.

Faunce, P. S. (1990). Self-care and wellness of feminist therapists. In H. Lerman and N. Porter (Eds.), *Feminist Ethics in Psychotherapy*, pp. 123-130. Springer: NY.

Feminist Therapy Institute Code of Ethics, 1999.

Fivush, R. (1997). *Feminist perspectives on the development of autobiographical memory.* Paper presented at the Engendering Rationalities, Eugene, Oregon.

Freyd, J. J. (1996). Betrayal trauma: The logic of forgetting childhood abuse. Cambridge, MA, USA: Harvard University Press.

Freyd, J. J. (1997). Violations of power, adaptive blindness and betrayal trauma theory. *Feminism & Psychology*, 7 (1), 22-32.

Gatens, M. (1991). Feminism and philosophy: Perspectives on difference and equality. Cambridge, England: Polity Press.

Griscom, J. L. (1992). Women and power: Definition, dualism, and difference. *Psychology of Women Quarterly*, 16 (4), 389-414.

Heyward, C. (1993). When boundaries betray us: Beyond illusions of what is ethical in therapy and in life. San Francisco: Harper Collins.

Hoagland, S. L. (1991). Some thoughts about "caring." In C. Card (Ed.), *Feminist ethics* (pp. 246-263): University Press of Kansas.

Kitzinger, C. (1992). Feminism, psychology, and the paradox of power. In J. S. Bohan et al. (Eds.), Seldom seen, rarely heard: Women's place in psychology. *Psychology, gender, and theory.* (pp. 423-442). Boulder, CO, USA: Westview Press.

Lerman, H., & Porter, N. (1990). The contribution of feminism to ethics. In H. Lerman & N. Porter (Eds.), *Feminist Ethics in Psychotherapy* (pp. 5-13). New York: Springer Publishing Company, Inc.

Lerman, H., & Rigby, D. N. (1990). Boundary violations: Misuse of the power of the therapist. In H. Lerman, N. Porter et al. (Eds.), Feminist ethics in psychotherapy. (pp. 51-59). New York, NY, USA: Springer Publishing Co, Inc.

Lips, H. M. (1994). Female powerlessness: A case of 'cultural preparedness?' In H. L. Radtke, H. J. Stam et al. (Eds.), Power/gender: Social relations in theory and practice. Inquiries in social construction. (pp. 89-107). London, England UK: Sage Publications, Inc.

Lott, D. A. (1999). In session: The bond between women and their therapists. New York: W.H. Freeman and Company.

Marecek, J., & Kravetz, D. (1998). Power and agency in feminist therapy. In I. B. Seu, M. C. Heenan et al. (Eds.), Feminism and psychotherapy: Reflections on contemporary theories and practices. Perspectives on psychotherapy. (pp. 13-29). Thousand Oaks, CA, USA: Sage Publications, Inc.

McCarthy, W. C., & Frieze, I. H. (1999). Negative aspects of therapy: Client perceptions of therapists' social influence, burnout, and quality of care. *Journal of Social Issues, 55* (1), 33-50.

Miller, C. L., & Cummins, G. (1992). An examination of women's perspectives on power. *Psychology of Women Quarterly, 16,* 415-428.

Newman, L. S., Duff, K. J., & Baumeister, R. F. (1997). A new look at defensive projection: Thought suppression, accessibility, and biased person perception. *Journal of Personality & Social Psychology, 72* (5), 980-1001.

Pennebaker, J. W. (1997). Writing about emotional experiences as a therapeutic process. *Psychological Science, 8* (3), 162-166.

Peterson, M. R. (1992). At personal risk: Boundary violations in professional-client relationships. New York: Norton.

Powell, W. E. (1994). The relationship between feelings of alienation and burnout in social work. *Families in Society, 75* (4), 229-235.

Riger, S. (1993). What's wrong with empowerment. *American Journal of Community Psychology, 21* (3), 279-292.

Sagrestano, L. M. (1992). Power strategies in interpersonal relationships: The effects of expertise and gender. *Psychology of Women Quarterly, 16* (4), 481-495.

Sagrestano, L. M. (1992). The use of power and influence in a gendered world. *Psychology of Women Quarterly, 16* (4), 439-447.

Sampson, E. E. (1993). Identity politics: Challenges to psychology's understanding. *American Psychologist,* 1219-1230.

Shange, N. (1987). Pages for a friend. Ridin' the moon in Texas. New York: St. Martin's Press. (pp. 33-34).

Siegel, R. J. & Larsen, C. (1990). the ethics of power differentials. In Lerman, H. and Porter, N. (Eds.), *Feminist Ethics in Psychotherapy,* NY: Springer, pp. 41-42.

Unger, R. K. (1986). Looking toward the future by looking at the past: Social activism and social history. *Journal of Social Issues, 42* (1), 215-227.

Veldhuis, C. B., & Freyd, J. J. (1999). Groomed for silence, groomed for betrayal. In M. Rivera (Ed.), *Fragment by Fragment: Feminist Perspectives on Child Sexual Abuse and Memory* (pp. 253-282). Charlettown, PEI: Gynergy Books.

Wendling, T. (1999) Disciplined psychologists face few consequences. Plain Dealer.

Wyche, K. F., & Rice, J. K. (1997). Feminist therapy: From dialogue to tenets. In J. Worell & N. G. Johnson (Eds.), Shaping the future of feminist psychology: Education, research, and practice (pp. 57-71). Washington, D.C.: American Psychological Association. *Quarterly, 16* (4), 381-388.

Yoder, J. D., & Kahn, A. S. (1992). Toward a feminist understanding of women and power. *Psychology of Women Quarterly, 16* (4), 381-388.

Exploring the Rift:
An Intergenerational Dialogue
About Feminism

Natalie Porter
Dalia G. Ducker
Holley E. Ferrell
Laura Helton

SUMMARY. Four psychologists, two "older" faculty members and two "younger" students, met to discuss their perspectives on contemporary feminism. The dialogue was intended to give the older feminists an opportunity to listen to their younger colleagues. A consciousness-raising group format with some planned questions was used. The report focuses on the younger women's thoughts and experiences. Among the topics touched on are: stereotypes of feminism, divisions among feminists, women's sexuality, political activism, sexual harassment, speaking out in graduate school, feminism in popular culture, and collaboration among feminists. The younger feminists articulated the need for more mentoring and support and questioned whether older feminists have been willing to see the goals and values of feminism adapted to keep pace with ever-changing societal contexts. *[Article copies available for a fee from The Haworth Document Delivery Service: 1-800-342-9678. E-mail address: <getinfo@haworthpressinc.com> Website: <http://www.HaworthPress.com> © 2001 by The Haworth Press, Inc. All rights reserved.]*

Natalie Porter, Dalia G. Ducker, Holley E. Ferrell, and Laura Helton are affiliated with California School of Professional Psychology, Alliant University.

Address correspondence to: Natalie Porter, CSPP/Alliant University, 2728 Hyde Street, Suite 100, San Francisco, CA 94109.

[Haworth co-indexing entry note]: "Exploring the Rift: An Intergenerational Dialogue About Feminism." Porter, Natalie et al. Co-published simultaneously in *Women & Therapy* (The Haworth Press, Inc.) Vol. 23, No. 2, 2001, pp. 57-78; and: *The Next Generation: Third Wave Feminist Psychotherapy* (ed: Ellyn Kaschak) The Haworth Press, Inc., 2001, pp. 57-78. Single or multiple copies of this article are available for a fee from The Haworth Document Delivery Service [1-800-342-9678, 9:00 a.m. - 5:00 p.m. (EST). E-mail address: getinfo@haworthpressinc.com].

KEYWORDS. Feminism, consciousness-raising, post-feminism

In this article we report on a conversation among four women psychologists who identify as feminists. Two of us are "older" faculty members, and two are "younger" students. The two faculty members, Natalie Porter and Dalia Ducker, initiated this conversation in order to learn more about what young feminists thought. Over the years we have noticed that few of the growing number of women graduate students in clinical psychology identified as feminists, and we hoped to understand why this was so. We also thought that talking with young women who could articulate their views about feminism and this rift would be a first step toward bridging it. We chose to use a consciousness-raising group format of sharing our experiences as a framework because we hoped that it would facilitate self-reflection and insight. In this context, we asked questions about topics we thought would be relevant, while being open to going wherever the conversation took us. We were there primarily to listen and to learn from our students.

We also saw this dialogue as an opportunity to mentor: to encourage young feminists to contribute their views to the psychological literature. Because we want to emphasize the younger feminists' perspectives, we focus on their voices in this report. The actual conversation occurred as more of a dialogue, with greater self-disclosure by all four of us, but we have chosen to omit some of the details. Thus, in order to set the stage, we began by sharing information about all of our personal lives, but we have included only the two students' contributions. Suffice it to say that there were some commonalities in the background of the two older women, both white women in their 50s. Both had strong mothers, experienced discrimination and sexual harassment, had engaged in political activism, and had early experiences with feminist psychology. Both had also participated in women's consciousness-raising groups, leading to an abiding faith in the power of coming together and listening to one another's stories.

BACKGROUNDS

Laura Helton: I'm 29 years old, and I'm what is considered "biracial." I never referred to myself as biracial until I moved to the San Francisco Bay area. Honestly, I am content to say I am a "halfie"–half Pilipino and half white. My dad, who is white, met my mother when he was stationed in the Philippines. I was born there and moved to the States when I was two.

I don't think of my feminist ideas as stemming from western feminism. They are more steeped in my mother's experiences as part of the Pilipino culture. My mother's beliefs were different from most other traditional Pilipino women of her day. My mother was considered quite independent and even had her own business in the Philippines during the early 1970s. At the time my mother's philosophy was that she didn't need to marry a man to better her life. Actually, a year before she met my dad, someone prophesied that she would marry an American. Her response was to say, "Why would I do that? I don't need a man to support me." But then she met my father, fell in love and left the Philippines for the States. Unfortunately, from my perspective, she got caught up in what she perceived as being the ideal American wife. She didn't work outside of our home for the first seven or eight years of my life and tried to keep the perfect house. Her children had to be perfectly clothed with perfect manners. She wanted us to be *American* children and only encouraged us to speak English. She didn't "push us" to learn Tagalog or any of the other three Pilipino dialects in which she was fluent.

Growing up, I knew my mother was strong-minded. She was outspoken, and she taught us to be outspoken. I was taught from an early age that education is key and not to build a life based on being supported by men. I grew up highly influenced by these values, but I didn't realize until much later that they embodied a feminist perspective. In the Philippines, my mother was considered radical for her ideas. In the U.S., with me, she focused on education, education, education. And she was strict and wouldn't let me or my four other sisters date at the age most girls started to date in Texas.

I grew up in Texas and still consider it my home. Texas culture is a world unto itself. Though women are encouraged to go to college, it seemed when I was growing up that the main reason for attending college was to find a husband. The joke at Texas Tech, where I completed my undergraduate studies, was that the majority of girls were working on their "MRS Degree." I would recount this to my mother who would say, "Don't listen to them. Career, career, career." I was pre-med at the time and strongly agreed with my mother that focusing on my career was most important. What I began to realize, however, is that in Pilipino culture, being a feminist includes having raised a family. The family comes first, so balancing career and family successfully is difficult. Although my mom pushed education, she also strongly believed in family commitments. As I've grown older, it has become more difficult to reconcile a career focus with a desire to have a family also. Yet I have recognized that having a family is important to both my culture and me. As I near 30, I realize I have roughly only twelve to fifteen more years to start a family. I find myself beginning to struggle with the career and family dichotomy and wonder how I will balance both worlds successfully.

At times, my undergraduate school seemed like one big fraternity and sorority. Many of the women seemed to me to be content to be viewed primarily as pretty attachments to the men. I did not encounter what I'd call "western feminism" there. I didn't really encounter it until I moved to the San Francisco area for graduate school. Wendy Stock's class, feminist approaches to sex therapy, was eye opening. Now, when I go home to Texas, I definitely discern a difference in attitudes regarding feminism there versus here. I have noticed that some of my female friends let a lot slide and take more of a submissive position in their interactions with others. I think they should "fight" more for what they believe. For example, one of my friends was passed over for promotion in favor of a man, when she had contributed more. I encouraged her to speak out, but her response was that her time would come. She appeared to resign herself to this outcome and not question it. When I return to San Francisco after a visit to Texas I sometimes think, "Wow, we're all living on the fringe out here." Then I remind myself, "No, women here are just more aware and willing to stand up for themselves."

Holley Ferrell: I'm a 25-year-old white woman, young compared to everybody else here. I think I was born a feminist. My father was career military, and I went to nine schools in twelve years. I don't know whether to attribute my characteristics to "nature" or "nurture," but I grew up as an outgoing and outspoken girl. I knew what I wanted and what I didn't want. Even at a young age, I would become very angry about the disparity in the gifts my younger brother and I would receive. His gift would be blue, and mine would be red. He would get the Star Wars sleeping bag, and I would get the Strawberry Shortcake bag. I was the bigger Star Wars fan. I hated Strawberry Shortcake, and I preferred blue. I remember feeling angry that I was forced to like certain things or be a certain way because I was a girl.

When I was in first grade I used to fight with my mom about my clothes. I wanted to dress myself the way *I wanted* to dress. She finally gave up. I also became aware of gender-based double standards growing up. I had a strict curfew as an adolescent, although my brother never had one his entire life. Even when I was 21 years old, they were strict and protective because I was a woman.

My parents have a tumultuous relationship and fought a lot while I was growing up. I witnessed my father putting my mother down and her feeling like she had to take it. At the same time, she conveyed to me, "Don't depend on a man and don't do what I'm doing." However, my mom did work as a nurse the whole time I was growing up. I considered her a role model when it came to working and education. My upbringing had the same mixed messages others here are describing. On the one hand, my parents would allow me to "be myself" and tolerate my violating certain social expectations. On the other hand, each of them had a difficult time breaking from those same social and gender role expectations.

I think I first became conscious of women's issues more broadly when I was in college. I started to recognize that the problems of my female friends were not just related to their individual contexts but to being female. I observed them being treated poorly, spoken down to, and insulted by boyfriends and male professors. I went to a very competitive university, which made it even more difficult.

I became aware of domestic violence in a societal context while I was in a sorority, which was part of a really dysfunctional system. It seemed to me that a lot of self hate was going on in the sororities–excessive drinking, unprotected sex, women allowing themselves to be dominated by guys. A friend was raped by a guy at a fraternity. She caught an STD that she'll have the rest of her life. She was suicidal about the rape, but she would not talk to anyone about it because she was so ashamed. She never received counseling.

Many women also seemed to be there primarily to find husbands. I became really angry about what I was seeing. I also got really angry about who my professors were. I didn't have any female professors who were role models for me. I remember feeling very alone and angry. I took a Psychology of Women class and really enjoyed it. It turned into a consciousness-raising group, as you described, Dalia, because women were speaking together about issues they had never raised before. I had never even considered them as topics to discuss. But the Psychology of Women office wasn't even in the academic buildings. It was located in the attic of an out-of-the-way house off campus. It obviously wasn't considered a central part of the campus. I hadn't even known about it until my senior year when I took that class.

I ended up writing an honors thesis, "Do today's women really have it all?" Basically, it was about home-career conflict. I had believed that as "today's women" we could do anything we wanted. We could have a career and children, and no one would judge us regardless of our choices. Then I began to question how does one really do both. No one has ever explained to me how to do both. I interviewed about 60 women about their views on home-career conflicts. I found that most everyone I interviewed either was planning to do what her mother or other family members did or had never really thought much about how they would balance their lives. They were just as confused as I was. The research project was an eye-opening experience for me. I ended up coming to CSPP because of the psychology of women emphasis area here. I didn't apply anywhere else, because I was starving for information about women's issues and feminism.

No one at my undergraduate school even uttered the word "feminist." They used the term "psychology of women." I first described myself as feminist here at CSPP. I would say that I was a feminist before then, but I had never described myself that way. Since I've been here I have taken several courses in feminist approaches to psychotherapy. They have all been incredibly eye-opening experiences for me. My heart rate goes up when I read the feminist literature and people like Laura Brown.

Natalie: I'm struck by the similarities of our experiences across the two generations. On the one hand, we are separated by 25 or more years. On the other, things haven't changed all that much.

Laura: I think society has worked "really hard" at not changing.

Holley: My family is very conservative, and the school I attended was very conservative. When I moved to the San Francisco Bay area someone asked me if I was going to become a lesbian. Another well-meaning person gave me an article from the newspaper that said to warn your daughters about the evils of feminism. He was serious. I thought it was funny.

VIEWS OF FEMINISM

Natalie: How similar do the two of you think your experiences are compared to other women graduate students here? You have emerged with a feminist awareness. Do you think you are typical or atypical? As we older feminists try to understand why there aren't many new or young feminists joining our ranks, one theory proposed is that there is no need for feminism anymore. We've progressed beyond gender distinctions. My own belief is that we've retreated into a more conservative era. What are your thoughts?

Laura: I think it depends on where you are. In my experience, though there are definitely liberal areas found in Texas, much of the state is conservative. In these areas, women's issues are rarely talked about. There, for example, if I were to point out discrepancies in women's earning power, people would look at me wondering where on earth I came from. If I made the same statement here in the San Francisco area, it would lead to a discussion of the factors involved, including the emergence of a new conservative era. People here would articulate concern about the bombing of abortion clinics, the attacks on *Roe v. Wade*, and other attempts to turn back what women have achieved over the past three decades.

Holley: I think both are occurring. Some take the successes of the women's movement for granted and aren't concerned. Others don't particularly care. Their attitude is more akin to "Let one of those diehard feminists worry about it."

Dalia: They think it isn't relevant to them?

Holley: Yes, I don't think they will get involved unless something does happen to them. If someone needed an abortion and that option was no longer there, she might get involved. Now it doesn't seem relevant.

Laura: I agree. The overt signs of discrimination aren't present now. What you described, Natalie, about being harassed while walking down the street, or you, Dalia, about not receiving a fellowship because you are a woman, probably wouldn't happen now, at least not in the same way. Discrimination has gone more underground. It is easier for someone to reassure herself that discrimination no longer exists than to recognize it and figure out what to do about it. I think young women are scared of being labeled as feminists, because they are all portrayed so unfavorably.

Holley: I find myself reluctant about speaking out about women's issues even though I've always been outspoken. If you asked me my opinion about women's issues, I wouldn't hesitate to give it, but I have never actively considered dedicating my life or career to addressing gender discrimination, raising political consciousness, or writing on feminist topics. I think that is because of the reputation of feminism.

The stereotype is that feminists are angry; they blame men for their problems. I see why that accusation exists, even if it is inaccurate. In one of my feminist therapy classes, we had a conversation similar to this: about "new" and "old" feminists. Some of the younger feminists pointed out how men are also affected by gender differences, having to adhere to rigidly enforced gender roles, for example. Some of the "older" feminists in the class said that our positions were hurtful and that they felt betrayed by us for this sentiment. The conversation became quite personal and emotional. We were trying to say that the previous generation of feminists were successful at articulating their concerns, making their anger heard, and achieving a certain type of change. But as young feminists, we believe that to change the system further we need to include both men and women in discussions about equality. We need to focus on how both groups are being negatively affected by the system. If men are the oppressors, they need to understand what they are losing by maintaining this system. We need to approach change from a different perspective. It hasn't necessarily worked the other way, and what remains is a bad image of feminists.

Natalie: So the issue for you is better coalition building?

Holley: Right.

Laura: And understanding that building bridges is most important now. In my experience, some women have been the staunchest anti-feminists. When I went to my high school reunion a couple of years ago, I felt the most disapproval for pursuing graduate school rather than raising a family from some of the women there. I received more support for expanding my horizons from the men there. So, I agree with Holley that coalitions with men are important, but I also believe that women need to learn to support one another. I am amazed at the ways we can tear one another apart over issues that should unify us. Of course, the media perpetuates this image by focusing on the disagreements and not the unity, but there is some truth to this part of our image.

Natalie: Are the negative stereotypes of feminists based on what they actually have done or are they manipulations by the media or conservative groups to discredit feminism and impede change? Isn't it easier to focus on feminist anger and unreasonableness than to address the issues? How much of this is done to drive away supporters . . . such as you?

Holley: I agree to a certain extent. I think what feminists see as the pursuit of equality is experienced by others as the threat of having to give up power and privilege. Similar to the fight against racism, if you recognize white privilege, you have to relinquish some of that privilege. However, I also think that trying to raise awareness from a different angle is important now. You need to show those who resist change how it could be better for them as well.

Natalie: What you're suggesting may be the evolution that occurs in many social movements. The first generation to embrace a particular belief may view the issue as a moral imperative–one should embrace a particular position because it is *the right thing to do.* The next generation may take a more pragmatic and less fixed position that takes into account that people act out of self-interest.

Laura: Another issue is what "traditional" feminism seems to leave out or ignore, such as having a family versus a career. You're not going to support a social movement if you feel you're going to be left out of it once you have children.

Holley: I want children; my boyfriend wants children.

Dalia: And somehow you've received the message that feminism can't accommodate this?

Laura: Most of my friends, particularly those in Texas, have kids. Some are in relationships where the man is definitely in charge, but others are in more equal relationships. Yet, it does not appear to me that either group considers women's issues relevant to their goals or lives. I think this is particularly true for my friends from ethnic backgrounds, where the stereotype is that "real feminists don't have children and families." In Pilipino culture I think this premise keeps some women from even exploring what "western feminism" does mean. I feel they may believe that it will not be supportive of deeply held roles and customs such as valuing family over career.

Natalie: I think that you are describing one of the aspects of feminism, particularly of early feminism, that has had the most difficult image problem. The image that feminism only speaks to and for privileged white women who want the goals of feminism to be almost exclusively independence and self-fulfillment. This form of feminism doesn't speak to women from collective cultures who value their communality, particularly if one of the messages is the devaluation of motherhood. I don't think that feminists have been the only, or even the primary, group to hold women who have stayed at home in contempt, but some of us have been guilty of this attitude, and we have been blamed for it all.

Dalia: I remember in my second consciousness-raising group, the one that had a mix of women who worked at home and graduate students, one student commented to the homemakers that our experiences were very different: we, the students, were using our brains all day long, while they, the homemakers, were using only their hands. I was astonished by such a parochial view and discouraged by how wide the gap was.

Natalie: Living in an agricultural state helped me to understand what you're describing, Laura, as a type of equality in ethnic cultures. Although the average citizens were not supportive of feminism, their interactions with each other seemed to lack the contempt I observed in more urban and suburban areas for women's roles. When both the man and the woman were rising at 5 a.m. to milk the cows and be involved in physical labor all day, a sense of respect and equality seemed to develop even when many of the tasks were gender-specific. This respect and sense of shared goals contrasted for me with the more affluent suburban life where the "what did *you* do all day?" contempt seemed to permeate relationships.

Laura: Again, this is an area where I found women to be highly judgmental. My oldest sister and her husband decided she would stay at home until her youngest child was in kindergarten. This was important to both of them, even though my sister was college educated. She has reported that she has felt scorned on several occasions by working women because she is not working outside the home. Some have even expected her to take care of their children as well, because after all, she is home anyway "without all that much to do." She felt most diminished in this role by other women.

Holley: I think that the observation that we've bred a culture of individualists is important. People in this culture, at least white middle class people, are very individualistic. If their individual lives are going okay they aren't concerned about others. As young women we are not becoming active because we are concerned with our own education and career goals. We're also focused on our relationships and starting families. We have not been raised to think politically.

My 65-year-old aunt was complaining to me that members of my generation are not patriotic and don't seem concerned with the affairs of the country. I replied that we have not been challenged in these areas. We have been raised by our parents to think that we can be whatever we want to be. We've never had to stop and think, "Gosh, we might have to defend the country, or gosh, I might have to fight for the right to choose an abortion." It has all been handed to us already. Even the feminist literature has been handed to us.

Laura: In the Pilipino culture, individualism is not a primary value. It is a collective culture. I was raised to believe the family unit was the most important thing in one's life. Family means not only the nuclear unit, but also includes members of the extended family and even friends.

Natalie: Maybe one of the disconnects between ethnic women and white women is that ethnic women can't survive by living so individualistically or apolitically.

Laura: Perhaps one of the reasons women I know feel left out of the feminist world is this individualism. We don't talk about "me" or "what

I need," but "what does my family need?" When they hear the term "feminism" they don't hear that connections to the family are possible.

STRENGTHS AND PROBLEMS OF FEMINISM

Natalie: What do you think some of the strengths and successes of feminism have been? What have some of the problems been?

Holley: There have been several important contributions. The reduced emphasis of gender in our society is one. It used to be that gender was *the* defining characteristic. Girls don't have to play with Strawberry Shortcake instead of Star Wars if they don't want to. Women can challenge the stereotypes. It is now acceptable to challenge certain behaviors or assumptions. There is more emphasis on equality and fairness, and people are more aware of what is not okay in speech or behavior.

Laura: I started to add that there are an increasing number of women working outside of the home, but I am unclear about whether this is a feminist development or an economic necessity.

Dalia: Choices about child bearing have changed with birth control. The need to plan what you would do if you got pregnant is less a theme for many women now.

Holley: Women now have a voice. We've been taught by our foremothers to question things, "Is this right? Is this fair? Is this the way it should be?" I have learned to question everything I see and everything I read. I question the psychotherapy techniques that are presented to me. Unfortunately, when I question my feminist foremothers, I feel like I've hurt some of their feelings. But I am doing what my feminist foremothers taught me to do.

When I question the social structure, I feel that women who don't assert themselves are proud of me. They tell me they are glad that someone is articulating feminist issues even if they aren't. I think the biggest contribution is that more women do feel that they have the right to speak out and question. I used to attribute my friends' lack of desire to speak out to their individual personalities and the way their families raised them. I didn't consider that it had anything to do with the larger context of being women.

Laura: Historically, I think about the hundreds of years that women have been treated like cattle, given to the highest bidder. Eighteen-year-olds were given to 60-year-old men for breeding. I can't fathom that we didn't have the right to vote until the twentieth century. Control of our bodies and childbearing through the birth control pill were significant developments. So was the increase in educational and career oppor-tunities. I recognize how glad I am to live in this era, after these changes. Women's sexuality is still one area that needs a lot of improvement. You can say "penis" all day, but "vagina" is still a taboo. The double standard remains around women having more than one sexual partner, using "raunchy" language, or meeting their own sexual needs. You are encouraged to seek sexual experience, but women who do so are still "sluts." Again, I find that other women are often the most critical of women who want to be more openly sexual. In the counseling I did with adolescent girls, I found that they know little about their bodies, much less what their body parts, particularly their genitals, were.

Natalie: You've hit on a controversial issue for many feminists. In our generation of feminists, sexual self-determination was an important theme for many. You may only be aware of this from caricatured im-ages of feminists, but in consciousness-raising groups, women strove to claim their bodies through group self-examination and discussion. How-ever, as you know, women are also on the receiving end of sexual vio-lence–rape, sexual abuse, sexual harassment. Forging a movement that discourages sexual violence while promoting sexual freedom has been difficult and certainly misunderstood. The consistency is clear to femi-nists–we are claiming the right to control our own sexuality–but lost on the public. It is satirized by the media and vilified by the right.

Dalia: I still remember the first time I talked to women about sex. It happened in my first consciousness-raising group. Before that, I never would have discussed my sexuality with a friend. I wouldn't have re-lated feminism to these conversations, but I see your point. Has femi-nism become almost puritanical?

Natalie: My guess is that puritanical values would be attributed to feminism more often than values of sexual freedom, particularly for heterosexual women. Lesbian women seem to have made more strides in defining and pursuing their own sexuality. What do you "young" femi-nists think?

Holley: Intellectually, I affirm our right to be agentic in our sexuality. Personally I find I'm scared to be agentic even though in other domains of my life I'm not afraid to ask for what I want. I wonder whether I am afraid of having that much power, whether I've been taught to believe that I'm not supposed to have sexual power. As a result I've become in-terested in women's relationships with their bodies and their sexuality and in sex therapy. I want to promote women's right to be sexual and encourage their active participation.

On the other hand, I have also worked at a rape crisis center for 2-1/2 years and am very much aware of the extent of women's sexual victimization. As we were discussing sexual freedom I was thinking back to a report that stated that in a certain area of Africa, some men believe they can cure their HIV through intercourse with a virgin. Rapes of young women have multiplied. When I hear such accounts, I feel powerless to help or believe there is a way I can make a difference.

Dalia: Are you struggling with how to integrate the personal with the political in your life?

Holley: I think I am. It is hard for me to know how to make the personal political. As a young feminist, that is the question I'm being asked, "Why aren't you more political?" I feel a bit like I've let down the older generation of feminists. I'm not doing my duty.

Dalia: You don't think you're being political by taking the individual stands you've described?

Holley: Yes, I do. The people I encounter–my women friends, women peers, classmates–respond that they appreciate my statements and are touched by them. They report that they experience something about themselves that they hadn't seen before. I am proud of this activity; yet, working on the bigger picture, by joining a political group or starting a consciousness-raising group, feels overwhelming.

Laura: I think what you're saying goes back to being raised with these individualistic tendencies. We do have our opinions and when asked, we do stick to them. So we are political to a certain extent. But are we being political compared to the previous generation of feminists? That level of political action or commitment just isn't found in our generation.

Natalie: Not every feminist was a political activist in our generation.

Holley: That is the image.

Dalia: In my experience, we mostly talked to our friends, to our colleagues, to our students. Most issues were addressed at the local level. Political activism tended to focus on particular areas such as reproductive freedom, equity in the workplace, and legal issues.

Natalie: Political activists have always been in the minority, and that has been true of the women's movement as well.

Laura: But we grew up with the image of everyone being a political activist. They show films in school of the protest marches; we assumed everyone was marching.

Natalie: But the marches didn't happen all that frequently.

Holley: My father was a veteran of Vietnam, and he has always had negative feelings toward anti-war protestors. Growing up during the anti-Vietnam era and the feminist era, I heard about the protests as if they were occurring constantly, even if they weren't. They were affecting everyone's lives one way or another.

Dalia: Activism did seem easier then. There was a lot going on; students were organizing around many issues on college campuses. Activism was part of a climate of political change, maybe of culture change. Nonetheless, it did not occur all the time or involve everyone.

Natalie: And the activists were still in the minority. As much as we deify the '60s generation, Nixon won the election.

DISAPPOINTMENTS FOR "OLDER" FEMINISTS

Holley: I am curious to find out what disappointments the older generation have about the newer generation of feminists. I assume that you are upset that we're not politically active enough, but I don't really know what the specific issues are from your perspective.

Natalie: One thing that frustrates me in this setting is how often I see women not willing to take on a voice, stating that it is too "unsafe" to do so. I see women preparing for professional roles in unprecedented numbers, yet they seem more unwilling to take stands on issues than in the past. From my perspective, it is safer than it ever was. For example, frequently a student may only be willing to inform me about sexual harassment if I keep it confidential. My attempts to remedy these situations are often restricted by this reluctance. I also feel disappointed when I hear women students not taking interpersonal risks, such as during a discussion in a class on diversity, because they "don't feel safe." I think they are mistaking comfort level or lack of anxiety with safety. Lack of safety seems to mean that someone will disagree with them or disapprove of their position. For me, lack of safety means that you are in physical danger or going to jail or being ostracized by your family or the community. People of color don't have the luxury of safety. Suffragists fighting for the vote weren't safe. Gays and lesbians coming out in public aren't safe. But here, expressing an opinion in a class may be uncomfortable but it isn't unsafe.

Dalia: I've been disappointed by the lack of progress in our field. I think that because there are so many women students in psychology graduate programs like ours, faculty sometimes think that that's good enough, that we've done everything we can. They don't worry about including gender or women's issues in their courses, the curriculum, or clinical training. Women students seem to believe this too. They don't see any problems with what they're being taught or not being taught. I would think that they'd expect more.

The other disappointment I have is that the outcome of much of the feminist movement is that women now aspire to succeed in the same ways men have succeeded or to have what men in our society have had. I wanted women to change the fabric of our society, not just join the male power structure. For example, I thought that we could develop new, more integrated work and family lives, not just encourage women to be superwomen and do everything. I didn't want women to adopt the same materialistic and competitive values that characterized our culture.

Laura: Your generation did that. I think the outcome of the movement has been perverted in a way, used.

Holley: What you just said brings me back to my earlier statements about change requiring a different route. I think what happened was that with the anger came opposition. The desire to create a different system was interpreted as male blaming. The genders became very separate. It then seemed impossible for us to knock down the system, so the prevailing attitude became, "If you can't beat them, join them."

At 25, I am becoming increasingly aware that I have the opportunity to make choices about how I want to live rather than merely conforming to what I've been told about how to live. In having the choice to be what I want, I don't think of myself as choosing to do what men do.

Dalia: In my idealism, one of the things I hoped was that as feminist values spread there would be less emphasis on material success, and we would be less economically divided into haves and have-nots. I don't see that happening.

Laura: And a different model of success–without the repressed emotions. To get to the "top," you've got to be made of steel, at least that was the message I grew up with. I remember thinking, "I don't want to be as heartless as some of the women are portrayed, even their clothing is masculine." I didn't want success to mean that I had to relinquish all of my femininity to become a prototypical man. I didn't realize that the older generation of feminists was also disappointed with this outcome.

Holley: I want to return to Natalie's point about women who have been sexually harassed who want to let someone know but are afraid to take action. Even though women students are now in the majority, we still lack power as students. It is still a really difficult process. We may need that faculty member to write a letter of recommendation, and it is the professor's word against ours. I can't guarantee that the outcome of my complaining will not also be harmful, so I would rather just go on and try not to let it bother me.

Natalie: So, this is another area where the issues really haven't changed as much as I'd like to think they have. You don't feel protected, and the costs seem too great if you confront the harassment. I may be expecting too much from you as women students when the social structure has changed too little.

Holley: The other aspect is related to what Dalia said earlier about assuming that because most of the students are women, sexism isn't an issue. But it isn't true. I've experienced many sexist encounters in graduate school; I've been assigned offensively sexist psychology literature to read.

Holley and Laura: And we've had almost all male professors.

Natalie: I wonder whether most of the women students here find that the sexism of the theories or readings is addressed. Do you think women are feeling resigned about these issues or apathetic or don't see the issues?

Laura: Actually, I think all three. Some don't catch on to the sexism; others don't feel compelled to confront it, and then there are those who seem resigned to it.

REACTIONS TO FEMINISM

Dalia: What happens to the two of you when you raise an issue?

Laura: Well, it depends on the topic. I have seen some rolling of the eyes for some because they don't want to talk about the issue or are uncomfortable with controversy, and for others because they don't want to take the time to discuss something that is "off topic." The response is, "Thanks a lot, I want to get across the bridge before traffic, and you bring *that* up."

Holley: I had a professor discussing diagnosis, and I raised the relationship of certain diagnoses to women's oppression. The professor grew angry. He became visibly red in the face and accused me of pointing fingers at people. I was also very angry. Several women thanked me for my statements.

I believe that the future for feminism is more positive than we sound here. The people of my generation are evolving to be aware of these issues and to appropriate them in their lives. My peers, both white and women of color, and I reflect on and discuss these issues; we are less inclined to talk about them in class because we fear a backlash from the professor. By the time we're the faculty, it will be commonplace to raise these topics. People will be less afraid to bring them up, and as professors and mentors ourselves, we will consistently attend to these issues.

Natalie: Do you experience backlash from your peers as well?

Holley: I've never feared backlash from a peer because I feel on equal ground with my peers. It is their right not to agree with me. They don't have the ability to make my life miserable because they disagree with me.

Laura: I have peers who are far more concerned about the reaction of their peers than of their professors. They figure that there is only one professor, and they can handle that disagreement. Their concern is the judgment of their peers. They stay within the bounds of "politically correct" speech.

Holley: The make-up and climate of the class may have something to do with this. Also the personal awareness of the individuals. For example, in my Women of Color class, we disclosed a great deal and felt safe doing so. My own awareness is such that I've stopped caring what people think of my opinions; perhaps that is part of my the feminist awareness.

Dalia: One major difference between a more collective and a more individual approach to feminism is the support that consciousness-raising groups provided. We could use the group to help us analyze what had happened, help us deal with the pain, and then help us get back out into the world. I think it is virtually impossible to do this work without a support group. You can't be out on a limb with most of your classmates day in and day out without having a group that will validate and support you.

Holley: I feel I've been validated by the people who come up to me and thank me for expressing the "unsafe" in the class. Even people who are acquaintances, who I don't really know, approach me to say that I made a difference in the classroom by confronting an issue.

Laura: I agree that can be the result, but some individuals anticipate the negative outcomes, and their fear keeps them from saying what they want to say.

Holley: As a feminist I would want a group who are not afraid to say what they think. Part of what makes me a feminist is having the power to speak out, to say things others might not like. My idea of feminism is a woman who takes the power–she may initially feel fearful but she speaks out anyway.

FUTURE DIRECTIONS FOR FEMINISM

Natalie: What do you think some of the biggest shortcomings of feminism have been and where would you like to see feminism go?

Laura: I would like there to be more of a recognition that there are varying shades of feminism. There is a continuum of women who have different visions about the same situation. I know women who won't consider themselves feminists because they aren't politically or socially radical. I say to them, "You vote; you are politically aware about issues; you're a feminist. Whether or not you want to marry is not the defining issue."

Natalie: When you mentioned "shades" I thought you were going to speak about "shades of women."

Laura: That goes without saying–there definitely needs to be more of a focus on the needs and agenda of women of color. Feminism needs to be brought into the popular culture more, so that we can raise our children to value the word "feminist." Through the popular culture, you're going to reach members of the various ethnic groups in the country as has happened in music and in popular readings. We need to go beyond the feminist literature that you can only find in a feminist bookstore in Berkeley and take feminism out of the academic realm into the everyday culture. People will recognize feminism for what it is and assess whether and how it can contribute to their lives–whether they're male or female, young or old, white or people of color. People fear the unknown, and feminism has remained an unknown.

Holley: People are still alienated from feminism, in part because it seems like an intellectual exercise and in part because people are scared of it. Many people fear that feminism will take something away from them.

Dalia: When you suggest bringing feminism into the popular culture, I think of Madonna. Is she a feminist? People equate her with feminism, but it is hard for me to see her as one.

Holley: I've thought about how to create popular portrayals of feminists and want to explore how we could do that.

Natalie: The feminists who succeed in the popular culture are ones who fit another stereotype about women. So Madonna is popular because she is sexualized; she fulfills male sexual fantasies. Although, in her autobiographical film, she made it clear that she is in control of her sexuality, and that scared a lot of men. I've heard a lot of men with no feminist leanings adopt feminist language to disparage Madonna when I think what they really didn't like was her uncompromising attitude toward being in charge.

Laura: They were afraid of her power.

Natalie: Exactly. However, popular culture's version of a feminist is still a sex object who works at a high-powered job. It perpetuates the myth that women have to be everything, stunningly beautiful and a genius workaholic; typically, these women are portrayed as dangerous or cunning.

Holley: I think that is changing, and at least, the image of women is being questioned. I don't think all women in the media are sex objects any longer. Or, if they are, it isn't because they adhere to one standard of beauty. I think change takes time but that change is occurring. If my generation of feminists continues to question whether women have to be seen as sex objects, the next generation will be different. For example, Camryn Manheim (1999) of *The Practice* has written a book that basically says, "I'm fat; deal with it!" It is a bestseller on the main tables of every bookstore. She may currently be the sole celebrity with this message in the popular media, but she is impacting others who will join her ranks.

Let's take the negative image of Madonna because she is sexual. There are always going to be negative images of strong women, and society is going to be afraid of them. We already have the negative stereotype of angry feminists sitting around in their consciousness-raising groups, not doing anything. There is always going to be someone who puts a negative label on these behaviors. But, if you give young people an image of a sexually agentic woman who isn't shut up by being labeled a slut, or who can be successful as a scientist, or weighs 200 pounds rather than 105 pounds, they will grow up with these images as the norm.

Natalie: What are your thoughts about making feminism more accessible through popular culture?

Holley: There could be a book or biography series for junior high school girls about feminists, who they are and what they think. Perhaps they could develop a positive image of feminists from the beginning. They will still hear the negative stereotypes and criticism, but they will be better able to weigh both sides of the argument because of their exposure to alternatives.

BRIDGING THE RIFT

Natalie: So how do we build collaborations across the generations of women and feminists? I believe that one of most ingrained aspects of sexism and ageism in our society is the complete devaluing of older women. The last thing most young women want is to grow up to be like their mothers. If the last generation of mothers were feminist, then you can't identify with those values or with the older women who have them.

Holley: We definitely need intergenerational coalitions and collaboration.

Laura: I've thought about this for a long time. Women need to come together and forge ahead as a sisterhood that allows a continuum of beliefs and lifestyles and values and ethnic backgrounds. I do think of Madonna as an example of a feminist, even if not the conventional stereotype of one. She was able to bridge different races. She had little girls at young ages realize that they could go out and be outspoken and be seen as strong, confident women. She's probably one of the few women who has appealed to girls of different races and ethnicities. Her message has been powerful, "Look at me, I'm a woman, and this is what I stand for." I think women need to build relationships with one another as women within our generation as well as across generations. We would learn from both.

Dalia: Where do you think we've let you down?

Laura: I wouldn't say that you have let us down. You have laid the groundwork and given us the advantages we had growing up. A lot of change occurred to make that happen. What has changed has allowed us to pursue our own goals. We have become more focused on our individual needs and are less political as a result, but it isn't the fault of the older generation of feminists.

One of the issues for us is developing the motivation to come together. For example, I know people who are angered by the ongoing sexism in society, but I don't see more momentum to counteract the sexism. I don't think this generation has that motivation. I don't think the momentum is there. But, I don't know how to bridge the apathy and forge closer relationships.

Holley: One disappointment I have is that I feel "unled," although I don't blame anyone for this. I have read some great feminist ideas but have not gone beyond that. One of the reasons I like Dr. Stock's classes so much is that she is concerned about my development as a feminist. I've never had anyone feel that way about me. I've never had a woman professor who had the time or inclination to be my mentor, to ask me a personal question, to encourage me to be one way or another. One of the reasons I am so self-reliant is that I've never had anyone take me under her wing and help me figure out how to write a non-academic article or start a group or become political.

Older feminists can help develop this momentum. They can serve as role models and mentors. We have to learn from you–how did you develop your momentum? How did you deal with sexual harassment or sexism? Here the alumni association started a mentoring program. I called a prospective mentor twice, and she never returned the calls. She's busy; she's a professional with children, working the second shift. Women professionals are already taking on the weight of the world within their own professional and personal lives and within their families. How can they take care of the younger feminists and help them as well? It is a difficult problem.

Dalia: You make an excellent point. In a study I conducted several years ago, I asked women professionals if they had female role models. None of them had role models for doing what they wanted to do. They had to piece them together, using many different people in their lives. There is also research that suggests that women aren't mentoring other women professionally as much as men are. With the demands of their personal and professional activities, they just can't give on any more. I know that was a struggle for me while my family was young.

There is another aspect of this issue that has to do with being self-conscious about bringing my personal life into the school. If I mentor you and am open and personal, am I being too maternal and not professorial enough? I know this is based on an old-fashioned view of what a professor is, but I have felt that I shouldn't bring my personal life, my beliefs and history into the workplace.

Holley: That's interesting, because my boyfriend has a male mentor and they talk personally. A mentoring relationship is a full relationship. I'm unclear why you think of it as maternal.

Dalia: It has to do with my professional experience as a woman. I was hired at CSPP over 20 years ago because the school needed women faculty. There were three of us, and I was the only one who lasted beyond the first year. In the summer after my first year here, I had a baby. I came back six weeks later, and no one ever mentioned it. It was as if nothing had happened. I learned to detach my personal life from my professional life. They are two separate spheres.

Holley: Perhaps keeping personal and professional lives so separate is no longer necessary. I want to return to the idea of de-gendering feminism. I've had men in my classes who describe themselves as feminists. I think that anyone who is interested in mentoring feminists should be open to mentoring both men and women who identify as feminists. It's another way to reduce the split between men and women, to include male allies in the dialogue. There are men who sincerely want to be a part of the movement. When I am a professor, I hope to have a feminist mentoring group that includes any and all self-described feminists.

CONCLUSIONS

This process was illuminating and energizing for the four of us involved. The two "younger feminists" raised a number of issues that need to be addressed even if the "older" generation of feminists are uncomfortable or disagree with their perceptions. The realization that members of younger generations have been chiefly exposed to and influenced by the media's portrayal of feminists underscored the need for us to pay more attention to making feminism more accessible through popular culture. This process has prompted us to explore ways to re-establish networks for dialogue and mentoring.

Questions regarding how to make room for new feminist ideas and new leaders were implied throughout this process. These questions must continue to be addressed for feminism to remain viable. Feminism appears to have influenced subsequent generations of young women, although not always positively. "Older" feminists must seek ways to support the emerging views of their younger colleagues and students. Dialogue is key. We hope that this article can serve as a catalyst for that dialogue. As a text, it could be used as a starting point for discussion.

REFERENCE

Manheim, C. & O'Donnell, R. (1999). *Wake up, I'm fat!* New York, NY: Broadway Books.

The Mentoring Process
for Feminist Therapists:
One Trainee's Perspective

Jill Rader

SUMMARY. Empirical research and personal narratives highlight the important role of mentorship in the training of feminist scholars and therapists. This article explores what we know (and don't know) about feminist mentoring, particularly as it relates to the practice of feminist therapy. A personal narrative of one trainee's experience of mentoring in her development as a feminist therapist follows. The article concludes with suggestions for other feminist therapy trainees. *[Article copies available for a fee from The Haworth Document Delivery Service: 1-800-342-9678. E-mail address: <getinfo@haworthpressinc.com> Website: <http://www. HaworthPress.com> © 2001 by The Haworth Press, Inc. All rights reserved.]*

KEYWORDS. Mentor, feminist, feminist therapy, women

In these days of cyber-connectedness, support for feminist therapists and therapists in training can assume many forms and span all regions

Jill Rader is a doctoral student in counseling psychology at the University of Texas at Austin.

Address correspondence to: Jill Rader, Department of Educational Psychology, University of Texas, Austin, TX 78712.

The author would like to thank her mentor, Dr. Lucia Gilbert at the University of Texas at Austin, for her guidance on this article.

[Haworth co-indexing entry note]: "The Mentoring Process for Feminist Therapists: One Trainee's Perspective." Rader, Jill. Co-published simultaneously in *Women & Therapy* (The Haworth Press, Inc.) Vol. 23, No. 2, 2001, pp. 79-90; and: *The Next Generation: Third Wave Feminist Psychotherapy* (ed: Ellyn Kaschak) The Haworth Press, Inc., 2001, pp. 79-90. Single or multiple copies of this article are available for a fee from The Haworth Document Delivery Service [1-800-342-9678, 9:00 a.m. - 5:00 p.m. (EST). E-mail address: getinfo@haworthpressinc.com].

of the globe. I first learned of this publication on young feminists via Ellyn Kaschak's announcement over the Division 35 listserv. I responded to her invitation to participate because, as a developing feminist therapist who has a relationship with a strong feminist mentor, I have been able to experience, firsthand, how feminist therapists are "born." It is my conviction that, in the absence of curricula and clinical settings offering training in feminist therapy, mentorship is the primary vehicle through which the "torch" of feminist therapy is passed. Furthermore, this mentorship can have many faces, particularly with the access to others and to feminist resources afforded by the Internet. In this article, I summarize the literature on feminist mentorship and share my own journey as a feminist therapist in training. Based on this research and on my own experiences, I offer suggestions for other up-and-coming feminist therapists.

THE IMPORTANCE OF MENTORSHIP
IN THE DEVELOPMENT OF FEMINIST THERAPISTS

Research has consistently demonstrated that mentors are important for women's career development. Women with mentors report higher job satisfaction, a greater number of promotions, and higher incomes (Ragins & Cotton, 1999). Mentors are defined as "individuals with advanced experience and knowledge who are committed to providing upward support and mobility to their protégé's careers" (Ragins & Cotton, 1999, p. 529). According to Kram (1985), mentors serve two sets of functions–psychosocial functions, which foster the trainee's personal growth, and career development functions, which promote the trainee's development within the professional and organizational arenas. Trainees are not the only ones who benefit from the mentoring relationship. Mentoring is a two-way street, a mutually beneficial relationship between two people who like and respect each other (Gilbert & Rossman, 1992; Kram, 1985).

The literature indicates that women, who encounter more barriers to their professional development, particularly in nontraditional careers, may benefit most from mentors but may, unfortunately, have the most difficulty finding suitable ones (Bruce, 1995; Gilbert & Rossman, 1992; Ragins & Cotton, 1999). For example, in academic settings, female students are hard-pressed to find enough female professors "to go around," due to the disproportionately low number of senior faculty members who are women (Gilbert & Rossman, 1992). And aligning oneself with a male advisor can sometimes be risky. Gilbert and Rossman (1992) noted that more than half of all women have been sexually harassed during their working lives and that sexual contact has been reported by as many as 20 percent of female students in graduate psychology programs. Other problems with cross-sex mentor relationships are more subtle and reflect unconscious gender processes. In their review of the effects of gender on mentoring relationships, Gilbert and Rossman (1992) reported that male mentors may adopt a "father" role that discourages a female protégée's autonomy. Gendered interactions reflecting male socialization to assume authority and female socialization to defer perpetuate an unequal power dynamic in cross-sex mentor relationships. Indeed, gender plays an important role in the mentoring process. Gilbert and Rossman (1992) provide support for the claim that experiences of female protégées differ substantially according to whether their mentors are male or female. One study revealed that female protégées with female mentors report more personal attention from their advisors than those paired with male mentors (Ragins & Cotton, 1999). Ragins and Cotton (1999) theorized that the decrease in social interactions with male mentors might arise from the fear that the interactions would be viewed as sexual or inappropriate in some way. Gender also seems to affect the rigor of the mentoring activities. Same-sex mentors assign more challenging tasks to their protégés than cross-sex mentors (Ragins & Cotton, 1999).

Beyond these overt and covert inequities that occur on the individual level, the organizational structure of women's departments or workplaces can discourage effective mentoring. Because informal mentoring relationships are based on a mutual comfort level and judgments of competence between mentor and mentee, women may also be at a disadvantage in seeking out role models, due to perceived and/or actual gender inequities in their educational and occupational environments (Ragins & Cotton, 1999).

Despite the obstacles to mentorship opportunities, studies show that women are proactive in seeking out role models. A study of women doctoral students revealed that women strongly value their relationships with mentors, particularly if those mentors are women (Bruce, 1995). Similarly, Gilbert and Evans (1985) reported that female students sought out same-sex mentors more than their male counterparts and valued those mentoring relationships more. Furthermore, women pursuing role models may be most attracted to those mentors who demonstrate competence in both the professional and personal spheres. According to Gilbert and Rossman (1992), such mentors "may provide unique role modeling for their protégés by demonstrating that women are competent in many areas and aspects of psychology as a field and that women can be leaders in their field. Perhaps more important, female mentors also can demonstrate that competent and achieving women have successful personal lives–that they are real people who are able to enter into loving and caring relationships with lovers, spouses, and children" (p. 235). Therefore, they add, women mentors may offer a type of mentoring that male mentors cannot provide.

Research on the mentorship process for feminist therapists is largely anecdotal, presented in the form of personal accounts and narratives (Brown, 1995; Kimmel, 1989; Knowles, 1995; Sonderegger, 1995). The lack of quantitative research on feminist mentorship reflects feminism's commitment to context, as well as the scarcity of studies on women's career development in the mental health professions. One psychologist in training commented, "Volumes have been published on the subject of learning psychotherapy–the hows, whens, wheres, and whys of being a professional therapist. Yet there are few narrative accounts of young therapists' early experience on the expedition: what maps guide us, and how do we learn to read them?" (Lillich, 1997).

Accounts from feminist therapists suggest that there are many paths to feminist therapy, but all mention the larger-than-life presence of early feminist role models (Brown, 1994; Kimmel, 1989; Sonderegger, 1995). These models have ranged from literary figures like Phyllis Chesler (for her groundbreaking *Women and Madness*) to feminist faculty members, advisors, fellow students and therapists (Brown, 1994; Sonderegger, 1995). That much of the information on feminist therapist development is anecdotal is not accidental. Ellen Kimmel, former president of Division 35, wrote, "The earliest definitions of our field . . . all emphasized women's experience . . . we should attend to experiences phenomenologically relevant to women that are not stripped of their social context" (p. 133). In keeping with this feminist tradition, a narrative describing my own path to feminist therapy follows.

THE IMPORTANCE OF MENTORSHIP
IN MY OWN FEMINIST JOURNEY

The transformative power of feminist mentorship is striking in my own evolution from a conservative, heterosexual, Southern Baptist woman from small-town Texas to my current identity as feminist therapist in training, an out lesbian, and a third-year doctoral student in the counseling psychology program at the University of Texas at Austin.

My first feminist role model was Dr. Nancy Chinn, a literature professor at Baylor University, who insisted that her reluctant students develop an enthusiasm for women's literature, particularly works by women of color. Dr. Chinn's feminism was largely unsupported at that time. She was the lone feminist voice in a conservative department at a Baptist university during the Reagan era. The full impact of her courage and commitment did not hit me until years later. It was in Dr. Chinn's class that I first encountered Toni Morrison and Zora Neale Hurston. Although as a White woman of privilege, I could not wholly relate to the experiences of these amazing writers, I certainly shared with the characters a desire to create something outside of my own narrow existence. Reading Kate Chopin's *The Awakening* paralleled the beginnings of my own awakening to feminist power and expression. It was my love of literature, women's literature in particular, that led me into the writing profession myself. I majored in journalism and earned my Bachelor of arts degree in May of 1989. I then became a newspaper reporter in Texas and New York for several years. I married a man I had met in one of my literature classes at Baylor and worked while he pursued his PhD in comparative literature.

But reading and writing other people's stories began to feel limiting, as well. I wanted to be less detached, less reactionary, about people's lives and about my own. I again looked for a way to broaden my professional, intellectual, and personal horizons. I wanted to find a way to better blend my newfound feminism into my work and into my life. My experience as a woman married to a man also heightened my interest in gender relations and sexuality, which led me to reading works by feminist psychologists. While my husband finished a post-doctoral fellowship in Atlanta, I took undergraduate psychology classes and began investigating graduate programs.

I first heard the words "feminist therapy" in a theories course taught by Dr. Andy Walters, a feminist instructor and much-loved student advisor in the psychology department at the University of Georgia. That my first feminist mentoring relationship was with a man has given me a somewhat unique and optimistic view of gender relationships and the flexible nature of feminism and "who is feminist." During this time, I read an article entitled "Gender and the Mentoring Process for Women: Implications for Professional Development," written by Lucia Gilbert and Karen Rossman (1992). Little did I know that I would eventually enter the University of Texas at Austin's counseling psychology PhD program and that Lucia Gilbert, a professor there, would be my mentor.

The beginning of my mentorship relationship with Lucia, almost three years ago, marked the beginning of my formal training as a feminist therapist and scholar. I already had the passion, ability and drive to pursue a career as a feminist psychologist, but I lacked the tools. Through example and instruction, Lucia has helped me to acquire those tools. Her invaluable feminist presence in the department, as the Director of the Center for Women's Studies, and, eventually, as Vice Provost at UT, has universally inspired admiration and respect. Her commitment to the mentorship of students and young feminist faculty members, teaching, and scholarship has been intense and longstanding. I had the privilege of watching my mentor operate in a variety of settings, through our mutually beneficial work together at Women's Studies (where I worked on publicity), on Lucia's research team, and through several writing projects. I watched her receive much deserved recognition and awards for her efforts (she was the 1998 recipient of the Carolyn Sherif award). Her classes on the psychology of women and on gender and sexuality provided me with the theoretical and ethical framework I needed to guide my research, work with clients, and, ultimately, my personal vision. Her classes also stirred in me the courage to come to terms with my sexuality, and acknowledging that sexuality was going to mean major life changes. My husband and I processed this stunning development with honesty and compassion. We decided to end our marriage but not our friendship, and remain sources of support for each other today. It was certainly no accident that my "coming out" as a feminist, as a strong woman, and as a lesbian were parallel processes. It was through the development of my love for women's scholarship that I was finally able to accept myself, and to give myself permission to love other women.

I have learned that feminist mentorship and support can come in a variety of forms and from a variety of sources. Building a vibrant and intellectually dynamic support system has been instrumental in my training as a feminist therapist. I've gained much support from women's research (Laura Brown's *Subversive Dialogues* has had a profound impact on my clinical work), peers in my graduate program and in other departments, friends, and a national community of female scholars, linked by conferences and online discussion groups. These sources of support have offered encouragement, opportunities to collaborate, the chance to mentor others, and the pleasure of intellectual dialogue.

My participation in the Advanced Feminist Therapy Institute this past spring in Portland, Oregon, was a defining moment in my developing career. Fortunately for me and two other students, one from Portland and one from British Columbia, AFTI decided to open its doors to graduate students for the first time this year. I had the rare privilege of meeting and talking with women whose scholarship I have read for years. Building on the long tradition of feminist mentorship, AFTI members were very welcoming and generous to us "newcomers." I was thrilled to have the opportunity to discuss my dissertation, a process study on feminist therapy, with women who have laid the theoretical and clinical groundwork for its practice. For three days, AFTI enabled me to interact with a roomful of potential mentors, women who are thriving in their professional and personal lives. As I listened to them describe the challenges and rewards of maintaining private practices, providing ethical services, coping with managed care, living with a disability, publishing books, and managing lesbian families, I realized that I was encountering, simultaneously, role models in multiple areas that I had never encountered before, role models I have longed for without even knowing it. Their stories, commitment to feminism and ethical practice, and efforts to live authentic lives bolstered my confidence in myself as a future feminist therapist, scholar, lesbian, and woman. I look to the future with hope, vision, excitement, and the knowledge that I am in very good company.

SUGGESTIONS FOR FEMINIST THERAPISTS IN TRAINING

Based upon the aforementioned research and on my personal experiences, I am offering the following suggestions to other up-and-coming feminist therapists.

Understand that Managing a Feminist Identity Is a Challenging, Lifelong Process

The commitment to a feminist vocation is a complex and psychologically demanding process that may involve initial fears about wearing "the feminist badge." For example, there is a tendency for students to shy away from the feminist label (Klonis, Endo, Crosby, & Worell, 1997). This may be due to realistic fears about how others react to the term (Klonis et al., 1997). Established feminists, however, report using the feminist label as a means of social activism and self-affirmation.

Kimmel wrote, "Upon first mentioning to an acquaintance, be they social or professional, that I am a feminist, I often notice a widening of the eyes or a slight catch of breath. Seizing the moment, I add quickly that, since it simply means that I believe in the equal worth of the sexes, I'm sure they must be a feminist, too" (1989, p. 135). Kimmel surveyed members of Division 35 and concluded that the feminist label becomes an integral and inseparable part of one's identity, and that "this identity, over time . . . become(s) less dramatic, and less questioned or self-conscious" (1989, p. 143).

It has not been conclusively demonstrated that a feminist identity is detrimental to one's career development (Klonis et al., 1997). However, feminist professors of psychology report a dishearteningly high incidence of gender discrimination within their departments (Klonis et al., 1997). In one study, a whopping 97 percent reported they had experienced gender discrimination, though the participants did not link their feminist identity to the discrimination. The authors commented that feminist women are likely to have a heightened awareness of discrimination. However, feminism also seems to empower women to deal effectively with such problems; in fact, 81 percent of respondents reported that being a feminist was an effective coping mechanism (Klonis et al., 1997). Brown (1994) wrote, "I cannot imagine that I would have been able to survive in psychology had I not found feminism and feminist colleagues there from my very first month of graduate school; I cannot imagine working, thinking, writing as other than a feminist" (p. 94).

Seek Out Feminist Mentors

The research suggests that a mentoring relationship may be one of the most important factors in the career development of young women (Bruce, 1995; Dannells, Rivera, & Knall-Clark, 1992; Gilbert & Rossman, 1992). Therefore, the search for an appropriate mentor is of utmost importance, particularly in the early portion of one's career development. There is some evidence that one's connection to a supportive person has the greatest impact if that connection occurs early along the career path (Williams et al., 1998).

If possible, the search for a mentor should guide one's choice of programs, practicum settings, and internships. Researching faculty publications and class syllabi can provide a quick glimpse of whether or not there are faculty interested in women's issues. Once you've narrowed the search, visiting programs or internship sites is an excellent way to scout out potential mentors. For a list of feminist-friendly graduate programs, check out this Web page address: www.feminista.com/gradprograms. html.

Of course, one might not have the option of selecting training opportunities based on feminist mentorship, particularly if students are limited to a geographical area or to a highly specialized area of study. In addition, finding a mentor who explicitly defines herself or himself as a feminist may prove very challenging in some graduate programs and training settings. Finding a same-sex mentor may be only slightly less difficult. Recall that research shows that same-sex mentoring relationships seem to be the most beneficial for female students. However, locating a feminist and/or female mentor may not be possible. In these cases, students may seek out advisors who promote the empowerment of their students, seem accessible, and enjoy mentoring activities and/or teaching. Word of mouth from other students is a valuable source of information with regard to potential advisors. Above all, the student should seek out a mentor with whom they share mutual respect and a sense of personal safety.

If support is not available within one's program or department, one might have to explore support elsewhere on campus. For example, taking a class by a professor known to endorse feminist views may open up a mentoring opportunity.

Seek Out a Support Group

A peer support group is an extremely valuable resource for feminist therapy trainees, particularly if mentorship opportunities are lacking. Williams et al. (1998) have emphasized the importance of a social network in the career development of prominent female academics.

Allow yourself to be flexible and creative in how you define your support group. Your peers don't have to identify as feminist in order for you to support and inspire each other. However, anecdotal evidence from feminist therapists suggests that surrounding oneself with strong, active women is very valuable for one's development as a feminist scholar and therapist. One study of feminist attitudes and behavior suggests that you may behave according to the company you keep (Branscombe & Deaux, 1991). More specifically, feminist behaviors are far more likely to occur if one is exposed to feminist beliefs and attitudes.

The widespread availability of electronic mail, online discussion groups, online journals and Web pages devoted to feminist issues provides ample opportunity to meet and share experiences with peers in a national, even international, arena.

Take Courses Grounded in Women's Scholarship

Coursework in the psychology of women is the exception rather than the rule at most graduate psychology training programs. For example, according to APA's *Graduate Study in Psychology,* the definitive listing of graduate psychology programs, only four programs (out of more than 600) offer the psychology of women as an area of study. Feminist therapy is not even listed (APA, 1998).

The absence of curricula focusing on women and feminist therapy is unfortunate because studies suggest that taking classes focusing on women's contributions significantly and positively impacts one's development as a feminist. For example, female students who take women's studies courses are more likely to endorse feminist attitudes and to be more critical of research on gender differences, when compared to controls (Thomsen, Basu, & Reinitz, 1995). Stake and Rose (1994) demonstrated that women's studies courses change women's behaviors, as well as their attitudes. After taking classes in women's studies, these women engaged in more feminist activism and reported changes in how they related to others. Furthermore, these behavioral changes remained at a nine-month follow-up (Stake & Rose, 1994).

Attend Conferences

My experience at the 2000 AFTI was a defining moment in my development as a feminist therapist. Without such opportunities to connect with other feminists in the field, the feminist student may feel "alone in the wilderness," particularly if she is working without the benefit of a mentor or support system.

Conferences, especially those such as AFTI or the annual meeting for the Association for Women in Psychology, present wonderful opportunities to find new role models and peers who share similar interests and values. Such conferences are also, of course, the sites for cutting edge research by women. Attending them simultaneously creates a sense of awe at the breadth and sophistication of feminist research, while demystifying the daunting process of presenting one's research. The hope is that developing feminist therapists leave such conferences with renewed excitement and commitment, as well as budding confidence in their own ability to join the intellectual fray.

Contribute to the Research and Visibility of Feminist Therapy

Laura Brown, in her keynote address at the 2000 AFTI, called for an increase in scholarship on feminist therapy (Brown, 2000). Outcome studies, she said, are particularly needed in order to promote the visibility, credibility, and continued growth of feminist therapy. Several members of AFTI also mentioned the need to better connect with newer generations of feminist therapists (e.g., by continuing to open the Institute to graduate students and by creating a Web page).

Joining the scholarship efforts of other feminist therapists serves multiple functions. First, it adds to the body of research in an area of counseling and psychotherapy that is still considered "fringe" by some. As Brown (2000) asserted, more research efforts are needed in order for feminist therapy to assume its rightful place in training programs and counseling settings. Demonstrating its efficacy is also crucial to the continued survival of its practice, particularly in these times of managed care and reduced therapist autonomy. Second, scholarly activity by feminist therapists increases the visibility of research by and about women. Women's scholarship and the psychological functioning of women have historically been excluded in the psychological literature. Finally, research efforts promote one's career development and help ensure that the noble tradition of feminist mentoring will continue for generations to come.

REFERENCES

American Psychological Association. (1998). *Graduate study in psychology.* Washington, DC: American Psychological Association.

Branscombe, N. R., & Deaux, K. (1991). Feminist attitude accessibility and behavioral intentions. *Psychology of Women Quarterly, 15,* 411-418.

Brown, L. S. (2000, April). *What we've learned in 30 years of feminist therapy: Making the political practical.* Paper presented at the meeting of the Advanced Feminist Therapy Institute, Portland, OR.

Brown, L. S. (1995). Notes of a feminist therapy "foredaughter." *Women & Therapy, 17,* p. 87-95.

Brown, L. S. (1994). *Subversive dialogues: Theory in feminist therapy.* New York: Basicbooks.

Bruce, M. A. (1995). Mentoring women doctoral students: What counselor educators and supervisors can do. *Counselor Education & Supervision, 35,* 139-149.

Dannells, M., Rivera, N. L., & Knall-Clark, J. E. (1992). Potentials to meet and promises to keep: Empowering women through academic and career counseling. *College Student Journal, 26,* 236-243.

Gilbert, L. A., & Evans, S. (1985). Dimensions of same-gender student-faculty role-model relationships. *Sex Roles, 12,* 111-123.

Gilbert, L. A., & Rossman, K. (1992). Gender and the mentoring process for women: Implications for professional development. *Professional Psychology: Research and Practice, 23* (3), 233-238.

Kimmel, E. B. (1989). The experience of feminism. *Psychology of Women Quarterly, 13,* 133-146.

Klonis, S., Endo, J., Crosby, F., & Worell, J. (1997). Feminism as life raft. *Psychology of Women Quarterly, 21,* 333-345.

Knowles, J. (1995). Enlightened, empowered, and enjoying it! *Women & Therapy, 17,* 291-299.

Kram, K. E. (1985). *Mentoring at work: Developmental relationships in organizational life.* Glenview, IL: Scott Foresman.

Lillich, S. E. (1997). Joining the expedition: Journal of a therapist-in-training. *Women & Therapy, 20,* 27-33.

Ragins, B. R., & Cotton, J. L. (1999). Mentor functions and outcomes: A comparison of men and women in formal and information mentoring relationships. *Journal of Applied Psychology, 84* (4), 529-550.

Sonderegger, T. B. (1995). Count me in. *Women & Therapy, 17,* 459-467.

Stake, J. E., & Rose, S. (1994). The long-term impact of women's studies on students' personal lives and political activism. *Psychology of Women Quarterly, 18,* 403-412.

Thomsen, C. J., Basu, A. M., & Reinitz, M. T. (1995). Effects of women's studies courses on gender-related attitudes of women and men. *Psychology of Women Quarterly, 19,* 419-426.

Williams, E. N., Soeprapto, E., Like, K., Touradji, P., Hess, S., & Hill, C. E. (1998). Perceptions of serendipity: Career paths of prominent academic women in counseling psychology. *Journal of Counseling Psychology, 45* (4), 379-389.

Feminism's Third Wave:
Surfing to Oblivion?

Lisa Rubin
Carol Nemeroff

SUMMARY. "Third wave" feminists, raised in the wake of an established feminist movement as well as a strong anti-feminist backlash, are beginning to define their own feminist agenda. "Third wave" feminists are exploring the contradictions in their lived experience as feminists, and examining the intersection of feminism with their other identities. Young feminists' self-expression has been characterized (by feminists and non-feminists) as "self-obsessed" and "divorced from matters of public purpose" (Bellafante, 1998, p. 57 & 60). In this essay, we provide an alternative view of "third wave" expression, seeing young feminists' honesty in their struggles with various identities as a resurgence of grassroots activism; a return to "the personal." In this essay, we call for an inter-generational dialogue between second and third wave feminists, and encourage feminist therapists to support and validate young feminists. *[Article copies available for a fee from The Haworth Document Delivery Service: 1-800-342-9678. E-mail address: <getinfo@haworthpressinc.com> Website: <http://www.HaworthPress.com> © 2001 by The Haworth Press, Inc. All rights reserved.]*

Lisa Rubin is a doctoral student in clinical psychology at Arizona State University. Her research focuses on feminist identity and body image among young women.

Carol Nemeroff, PhD, is Associate Professor of Clinical Psychology at Arizona State University. A major focus of her research is women's health, including body image and magico-moral thinking about food and eating.

Address correspondence to: Lisa Rubin, Arizona State University, Department of Psychology, P.O. Box 871104, Tempe, AZ 85287-1104 (E-mail: lisa.rubin@asu.edu).

Supported in part by an APA Division 35 Hyde Research Grant and a grant from the Intergroup Relations Center of Arizona State University, both awarded to the first author.

[Haworth co-indexing entry note]: "Feminism's Third Wave: Surfing to Oblivion?" Rubin, Lisa, and Carol Nemeroff. Co-published simultaneously in *Women & Therapy* (The Haworth Press, Inc.) Vol. 23, No. 2, 2001, pp. 91-104; and: *The Next Generation: Third Wave Feminist Psychotherapy* (ed: Ellyn Kaschak) The Haworth Press, Inc., 2001, pp. 91-104. Single or multiple copies of this article are available for a fee from The Haworth Document Delivery Service [1-800-342-9678, 9:00 a.m. - 5:00 p.m. (EST). E-mail address: getinfo@haworthpressinc.com].

KEYWORDS. Feminism, young women, third wave, body image

Gaining weight and pulling my head out of the toilet was the most political act I ever committed. (Abra Fortune Chernik, 1995, p. 81)

My body is fucking beautiful, and every time I look in the mirror and acknowledge that, I am contributing to the revolution. (Nomy Lamm, 1995, p. viii)

Over the past few months, we have been conducting focus groups with young feminist women about body and beauty. Feminism transformed how Lisa (a graduate student in Clinical Psychology) understood her own struggles with her body, as had happened for Carol (her graduate advisor) a generation earlier. We were curious if this experience was common to other young feminists as well. We decided to run these groups because we wanted a space for women to share their body narratives with one another, to speak about what they have been through, where they have come to, and where they still wish to go in terms of their relationship with their bodies.

Though the purpose of this project was not specifically to examine feminist concerns among the "third wave" of feminists, it became clear that any analysis would be incomplete if it did not consider the circumstances in which these women had come to know feminism, including the institutionalization of feminism as a discipline in the academy, and the ongoing backlash against it.[1] However, as we try to describe the influences that have shaped the lives of young feminists, we continue to struggle with who they are, and why we feel we can speak about, or on behalf of, this diverse group of women. However, we feel that (we) young feminists are eager to have our voices heard, and that it is of the utmost importance that (we) as psychologists "Listen Up."

EMBODIED CONTRADICTIONS OF FEMINISM'S THIRD WAVE

This is undoubtedly a confusing time to become a feminist. Young women today are growing up during a cultural backlash, and gender inequality is viewed as something of the past. In fact, the popular press has recently pronounced the death of feminism (see Bellafante, 1998). At the same time, with the establishment of women's studies programs on college campuses across the nation, feminist theory is even more accessible and perhaps more "sophisticated" than ever before.

We believe the conflicting messages arising from this particular socio-historical moment are embodied in the types of feminist expression emerging from the new wave of feminists. Young feminists are speaking up about the contradictions they experience as young women and as feminists in a manner informed by postmodern, multicultural, and queer theories.[2] This "third wave" is creating its own feminist agenda, one which both overlaps with and departs from traditional feminism. Third wave feminists aim to disrupt, confuse, and celebrate current categories of gender, sexuality, and race. These categories are typically both defined by, and resisted and/or celebrated through, body and physical appearance; therefore, in this essay we explore the personal and political aspects of third wave feminism primarily by examining young women's relationships with their bodies.

Amelia Richards remarks that "body image may be the pivotal third wave issue–the common struggle that mobilizes the current feminist generation" (1998, p. 196). Whether body image is *the* issue for young feminists, or just one important part of the third wave feminist "agenda," it is certainly an issue that young women are excited to speak about. Having had their consciousness raised in the academy, rather than through consciousness-raising groups that build on one's lived experience (as their feminist foremothers did), third wavers are crying out for space in which to examine their unique concerns as young feminists, the contradictions and ambiguities they struggle with in claiming a feminist identity. Despite current feminist theorists' emphasis on the diversity of feminist perspectives, many young women have perceived and are struggling with a normalized view of the "good feminist"–the woman who refuses to discipline her body and has learned to love her body and herself. Through our focus group discussions, the third wave essays we've read, and our own experiences as a young and a not-so-young feminist, we hear young feminists yearning to add their voice to the feminist dialogue.

CHARTING THE THIRD WAVE

Some young feminists have pronounced the dawn of a new wave, the third wave, of feminist activism. Whereas the term "second wave" served as a bridge between early feminist activities and ideas that lead up to the passage of women's suffrage in 1920 and the women's movement of the 1960s and 1970s, the pronouncement of the "third wave" is an attempt to distinguish it from second wave feminism (Bailey, 1997), as well as the backlash and/or "postfeminist" writings that came after (e.g., Katie Roiphe's [1993] *The Morning After: Sex, Fear, and Feminism*, and Naomi Wolf's [1993] *Fire with Fire*). Not surprisingly, not all feminists have embraced, or even given recognition to, this shifting tide. In general, young feminists have been characterized as overly critical of second wave feminists; their activities as not sufficiently organized or active enough to constitute a genuine movement (see Orr, 1997; Bellafante, 1998).

Rebecca Walker, co-founder of Third Wave (an organization for young feminists) and editor of the third wave anthology *To Be Real*, explains third wave feminists as doing "the difficult work of being real (refusing to be bound by a feminist ideal not of their own making) and telling the truth (honoring the complexity and contradiction in their lives by adding their experiences to the feminist dialogue)" (Walker, 1995, p. xxxiv). The personal essays in *To Be Real*, and other third wave texts, such as Barbara Findlen's *Listen Up: Voices from the Next Feminist Generation* and Ophira Edut's *Adios Barbie*, explore contradictions and ambiguities in young feminists' lived experiences, examining what these women find empowering, "irrespective of what is *supposed* to be empowering" (Walker, 1995, p. xxxvi). Through their narratives, many of these young women are resisting what they have interpreted as a monolithic view of the "good feminist," and in doing so, are achieving a deeper sense of self-acceptance.

For example, in her essay, "Close, but no banana," Anna Bondoc (1995), an Asian-American third waver, lays out what she calls her political sins against feminism. Bondoc states, "(1) I come from an upper middle-class family. (2) I'm not a full time activist. (3) I don't identify exclusively with an Asian-American community. (4) I love a white man. (5) I'm not angry enough" (pp. 169-170). She adds:

> Certain progressive people whom I've both met and, at times, emulated, focus so sharply on shaping themselves into perfect beings: color-blind, well-read, articulate people who can organize rallies, volunteer in soup kitchens, raise thousands of dollars for the good fight, and leap tall buildings in a single bound. (p. 170)

As her essay unfolds, Bondoc comes to "shed the 'sin' label" and reclaims each of these self aspects as part of her identity, describing them as "comforting, because I come to accept myself as a reality, not an ideal" (p. 171).

AN EXCERPT FROM OUR ONGOING
INTERGENERATIONAL DIALOGUE

Carol: Um, Lisa? I don't want to speak for the "second wave feminist establishment" or anything, but where is this monolithic view coming from? Having come of age in the mid 1970s, I personally interpreted feminism as my mother buying herself a "screw you" keychain, and learning to say "no" to my father; as my own belief that I could have any career that I wanted and be paid for it appropriately; and as my conviction that I do not need to be dependent on or submissive to anyone. Feminist ideology colored my teaching methods, my therapy approaches, my personal relationships including marriage and mothering. Yet I don't remember any monolithic movement where every one of my cohorts was offered plentiful consciousness-raising groups and a clear sense of activist purpose. When did second wave feminism supposedly become "monolithic"–and the property of academia?

Lisa: As young women learn the discourse of feminism in formal settings, many of us feel that because our "mothers" named and changed the nature of our oppression, we owe it to them, to ourselves, to live as "good feminists"; to love ourselves and believe in ourselves as they could not. What I heard from some of the young feminists in my focus groups, many of them women's studies majors and minors, was that while their consciousness had been raised, they continued to struggle with negative feelings about themselves and their bodies. For some women, there was a sense of shame, not only about their bodies, but additionally that as feminists, they had these negative feelings. It was difficult for them "to be real" and "to tell the truth" about personal feelings they had that challenged their feminist values. One focus group participant exclaimed:

I feel guilty for being aware [of my body], because I know that it's, it's trivial, and being a feminist I, you know I feel, oh, I shouldn't worry about that cause I know better. But I still, no matter what I do, it doesn't go away. It's always there.

And after participating, another group member remarked, "It felt really good to hear that other feminists have a hard time living the life of a good feminist."

Carol: So, are you saying that the preoccupation with body and self-image is young women's attempt to live up to the ideals that they perceive their "mothers" (both biological and academic) to have set out for them?

Lisa: Well, I think it's actually kind of the opposite–it's their preoccupation with *not* being preoccupied. Feminism has raised many young women's awareness of the economic and social profitability of women's bodily discontent. I see feminist consciousness as providing a means through which women can re-interpret their own sense of body dissatisfaction–if they experience it–understanding it as a manifestation of social injustice rather than the result of their own personal inadequacies. However, according to some of my focus group participants, when despite their awareness they continue to have poor body image, they feel like cultural dupes. This may compound the stress young women/feminists already experience about their bodies, and may cause them to remain silent about their own personal struggles.

Carol: As I understand it, young women are trying to take the next step–the step that many of their feminist mothers could talk about but not quite accomplish. A quote by Lee Damsky (1998) from *Adiós Barbie* comes to mind about her own mother, as she saw her during her critical, formative teenage years:

> I know that she doesn't think of herself as beautiful or attractive. I know that her body is a source of anxiety for her, not a source of power or joy. I'm puzzled by her insecurity. I wish she would snap out of it and teach me how to be a woman. I want a kind of power that my mother doesn't have. (p. 134)

Lisa: Yes, and I think third wave feminists are beginning to speak up about these contradictions. Nomy Lamm, a self-described "fat, sleazy, one-legged, anarchist dyke, and a total hottie" (1998, p. 82) writes:

> I've come to a place where I can honestly say that I love my body and I'm happy with being fat. But occasionally, when I look in the mirror and I see this body that is so different from my friends', so different from what I'm told I should be, I just want to hide

away and not deal with it anymore. . . . Would it be easier for me
to just give in and go on another diet so that I can stop this per-
petual struggle? Then I could still support the fat grrrl revolution
without having it affect me personally in every way. And I know
I know I know that's not the answer and I could never do that to
myself, but I can't say that the thought never crosses my mind.
(1995, p. 87)

These young feminists–Anna, Lee, Nomy, and some of my focus group
participants–are challenging myths of the "good feminist," however
mythical the reality of that image. These third wavers are courageously
breaking silences that prevent them from "being real" to themselves and
to others.

"THE PERSONAL IS (STILL) POLITICAL"

We think an important issue to address, given the critiques of young
feminists as "self-obsessed," "flighty," and "divorced from matters of
public purpose" (Bellafante, 1998, pp. 57 & 60) is whether third wavers'
self-reflections, their grapplings with contradiction and ambiguity, can be
viewed as political expression. Has feminism indeed "devolved into the
silly" (Bellafante, 1998, p. 58) or are young feminists accomplishing the
next step in forwarding the cause? What impact, if any, do their confes-
sional tales have on feminism as a movement and as a discipline?

What we see in these expressions of struggle with body and identity
by third wave feminists is a resurgence of grassroots activism, a return
to the personal in third wave narratives. While the women's movement
has broken through so many of the external barriers to women's full
participation in Western society, we feel that at this socio-historical moment the truest, biggest, and most crippling obstacles are internal. These
internal shackles facilitate the perpetuation of other, more external, barriers, as the following quote, by Marisa Navarro, a self-described "queer
Latina feminist," in her essay "Becoming La Mujer" (in *Adiós Barbie*),
starkly illustrates:

I'm tired of having my body picked apart by my father, being a
virgin but made to feel like a whore. I figure since I'm already
dirty, having sex won't make it any worse. . . . In bed, the boy
I'm dating pulls my hair and pretends to slap me to make his dick
harder. He calls me a slut and a ho'. I lie flat as a board, con-

fused, scared, and sexually unfulfilled. I let him fuck me without a condom, without birth control pills, nothing. My body is too dirty to be worth protecting against AIDS or pregnancy. (1998, p. 43)

Later in the same essay quoted from above, Navarro explains:

I thought racing to be part of the queer community would save me. I enlisted in the dyke world complete with uniform–short hair, overalls, cap on backwards and body piercings. . . . Now, instead of wanting to be the good hijita, I found myself trying to be a good queer girl and a good feminist. The role was just as confining. . . . The most political statement I could make was to look the way I wanted and not be ashamed of it. . . . . But that's what being a real *mujer* is all about. (1998, p. 45)

Or, as one of our focus group participants put it:

I . . . (believe) that the way for feminism to advance itself is just don't date jerks . . . . If women just, you know, don't date jerks, then men will figure out that, you know, if they're jerks, then they won't get any. You know? The world will be a better place.

How could a young woman possibly achieve this while immersed in self-doubt and self-loathing? Based on these types of quotes and accounts from multiple sources, and our own lived experience, we feel that the body focus of the young feminists, and especially their attempt to transform self-loathing into self-respect, is far less discrepant from the campaigns waged by their foremothers than it seems to those who approach it at a superficial level of analysis.

In an era in which women are bombarded with messages that they are naturally, inherently flawed–too young or old, too smart or not smart enough, too fat or not soft enough–self acceptance is indeed political, even if some aspects of what they are accepting seemingly contradict feminist theory. Though the form (personal narrative rather than group consciousness-raising) and content (examining, often celebrating, difference rather than seeking commonality) of personal expression in the third wave may differ from that of the second wave, we believe their functions are quite congruent. Rita Alfonso notes:

Even if third wave feminists perform their feminism in a way that may, in many cases, be *continuous* with (italics added) second wave feminism, these performances may not even register as feminist performances on a traditional, liberal feminist scale. (Alfonso & Trigilio, 1997, p. 11)

A major reason for the differences in modes of expression is likely to be that very bombardment against which young feminists (if not all young women) are struggling. One focus group participant put it plainly: ". . . but there's so much all around you that it's really to just keep everyday, reminding yourself, no you're ok, just cause you don't weight 100 lbs, that doesn't mean you're not the right person . . . [it's] a struggle." As technology and the electronic/video age have become central to our modern, consumerist society, images of "perfection" that could never be realized in an actual, healthy, female body, are everywhere. Airbrushing has given way to computer-generated composite images, and even complete fabrications. Visual representations of the "good" body lurk in magazine covers at grocery check-outs; unpredictably leap out of the large-screen high resolution TVs in our living rooms in the middle of the evening news; right along with ever more miraculous-sounding diet and fitness aids. Not only have expectations for achieving the "ideal body" increased, but this ideal form seems to be thinner now than ever before. This shift is clearly illustrated by a quote from the dieter's section of our B'nai B'rith Women's cookbook from 1968:

My chubby friend, your dream's come true,
We've added this section just for you.
If size eleven has been your desire,
Cut out the cheating, hubby sure will admire!

How much worse does a "normal" body feel for the young women of today subjected to signs boasting "come see our expanded selection of size 2's" on a casual stroll through the mall. "And what on earth," asks Carol, "is a size 0? What does it communicate to my 4-year-old daughter to speak of the ideal woman's size being literally nothing?"
(An excerpt from one focus group:)

Participant A: I don't know if you guys pay attention to magazines but, um, compared to Calista on Ally McBeal, there's Georgia, do you know who Georgia is? Do you know what size she is? What size do you guys think she is?

(One says six, one says eight.)

Participant A: One.

Moderator A: What?

Participant A: She's a size one. So what does that tell you about the sizes that people look like on T.V.?

(Someone gasps.)

Participant A: And then you gotta realize that the one that's the receptionist, Elaine, she's probably a normal [size], but ... she kind of looks big compared to everyone else.

Elaine, it turns out, is a size 4. Unfortunately, however much one may know, cognitively, that theses images are inappropriate, the aesthetic conditioning that seems to result from this bombardment is not so easily discarded:

Participant B: I think they look good, but the more I think about it, I'm like wow, that's really unhealthy, you know, she's probably malnourished. But at the same time I think it still looks good, I still think it's beautiful.

IMAGE: A WEAPON OF RESISTANCE?

As the pressure to achieve this "no body" body has increased exponentially, young women/feminists have attempted to rebel/resist by reclaiming their physical appearance as their own, often carried out through body piercings, tattoos, and fluorescent hair cut in bizarre shapes. Many young feminists use unconventional fashions and body adornment to resist symbolically the feminine fashions and consumerism that have long been considered one of the key sources of girls' and women's oppression. "In a society predicated upon the marketing of images, images become a weapon of resistance" (Ewen & Ewen, 1982, as cited in Nava, 1992, p. 163). Mica Nava (1992) describes the ways in which political groups often resist negative, controlling images by substituting alternative images and alternative ideologies (e.g., Black is Beautiful). Third wave feminists provide alternative images of femaleness, proclaiming that being "girl/woman" can mean being loud, being sexual, and being angry.

However, young women/feminists have been recognized by marketers not only as a target audience with discretionary dollars, but also as a new and highly marketable image that can be profitably exploited. The "image as weapon of resistance" when taken up as high fashion, suddenly becomes bereft of political significance. For example, ads for the Calvin Klein fragrance "One" connoted feminist/postmodern questions about the rigidity of gender and sexuality. While these ads clearly demonstrated the ways in which feminist postmodern theory has affected consumer marketing strategies, we doubt that most feminists would see such ads as a vehicle for promoting feminist consciousness. Many of today's "rebel youth" therefore find themselves surfing the edge of an ever-accelerating consumerist wave which constantly threatens to swallow up their political resistance strategies–if not their entire identity–into the undertow.

In our highly visual and image-centered culture, it should come as no surprise that image and identity are key issues with which young feminists are grappling. Learning to be true to oneself becomes an increasingly difficult developmental task in a culture in which pre-packaged identities are sold in malls and vintage clothing shops. We view third wavers' efforts "to be real," to air their personal dirty laundry even when it seems to contradict their political goals (e.g., "confessing" their struggles with body image while being part of the "fat grrrl revolution"), as an attempt to disrupt consumerist co-option. By seeking methods of resistance that grow out of their lived experience, third wavers avoid creating yet another idealized feminist image for their generation, and carve out instead a feminist space that can accommodate the diversity of their experiences.

IMPLICATIONS OF THIRD WAVE FEMINISM
FOR FEMINIST THERAPISTS

What can we glean from the foregoing that might help feminist therapists and mentors support the development of young women in general, and young feminists in particular? First and foremost, we think many of these young women are looking for spaces and settings *outside* of their classrooms–be they discussion groups, focus groups, therapy groups–to share their excitement and their struggles as they "try on" feminism and other alternative identities and ideologies. Young feminists are already creating these spaces, through Internet chat rooms and "zines," but many young women would likely benefit from options for negotiating and processing in "real-time" with real people in a way that these sources cannot fully provide. Young feminists/women need a different brand of consciousness-raising group which allows them to not only explore shared themes of oppression, but also learn to share, respect, even celebrate their differences. We believe feminist therapists are well positioned to help young women create these spaces. For example, feminist therapists working in college counseling centers or on high school campuses might organize free or very low-cost discussion groups. Along related lines, here at Arizona State University, the "Intergroup Relations Center" has created dialogue groups, called "Women's Story Circles," that are facilitated by graduate students from Counseling, Clinical, and various other programs. In terms of more traditional therapy settings, such groups would constitute suitable *pro bono* contributions for feminist therapists, and they could be integrated as well into formal psychotherapy for many of the current concerns that bring young women in for treatment, such as eating disorders, poor self-esteem, and depression.

Discussion groups could be included as a standard part of any professional conferences or events. At a broader community level, feminist therapists could seek out and attend those venues and events already attended and created by young feminists (e.g., coffee shops, youth conferences) and assist them in organizing both one-time and ongoing spaces for expanded discussion. This is not to suggest that feminist therapists should necessarily "lead" these groups. Rather, they can facilitate and support their organization by using their professional skills and credibility to help obtain space, funding, publicity, and so on.

Young feminists also need support and validation for the process from their feminist "mothers." We want to impress upon both second and third wavers the importance of intergenerational dialogue, to defuse the process whereby second wavers are increasingly cast by third wavers as monolithic and rigid, and third wavers as frivolous and self-obsessed by second wavers. We need to take a developmental perspective and understand that, whether or not one resonates personally to the voices of the third wavers, their concerns are real and a legitimate outgrowth of the second wave efforts. Young feminists' struggle for individualized feminist expression could not have happened without the collective movement of the second wavers to allow women to express anything at all. By the same token, the fourth wavers (or whatever they may come to be called) hopefully will have transcended these "self-obsessed" struggles thanks to the hard internal work of their third wave mothers. Mutual respect and a temporal perspective that follows feminism as it unfolds over time, through multiple generations and iterations, can only strengthen the movement. Mutual intolerance and failing to acknowledge the interdependency of the waves and their goals undermines feminism's transformative possibilities.

As feminist therapists, we can learn from our young clients too, as their struggles are not so different from our own. Feminist therapists have to resolve contradictions between traditional and feminist practice of psychology, including egalitarian versus hierarchical relationships between "doctor" and "patient"; the role of self-disclosure; and how to be genuine with our clients within the bounds of current ethical standards and while maintaining the therapy setting as a safe space for clients. Just as young feminists are trying to maintain their individual voices we also struggle against homogenizing influences in our profession, such as managed care limitations and therapy-by-manual trends.

Feminist therapists and academics, and "second wavers" in general, are in the perhaps uncomfortable position of having the power to legitimize or marginalize young women's efforts and concerns. Debi Morgan (1995) wrote, "young women are situated right at the margins of feminist theory because they are not actively involved in creating it" (p.133). We disagree. Yes, they may be writing from the margins, but Deborah Siegel (1997) reminds us that "the grassroots has always been a space for the production of theory" (p. 51). With Siegel, we think that theory is indeed being produced through the personal narratives of the third wave.

NOTES

1. This "epiphany" came to me (Lisa) during a discussion at the conference for the Association for Women in Psychology (AWP, 2000). I thank the "second wavers" in the group for raising many of these issues, and for encouraging what will hopefully be an ongoing, intergenerational dialogue around these issues.

2. This is certainly not the case for all young women, or even all young feminists. However, we believe this is a good characterization of the type of feminist expression that has been labeled "third wave."

REFERENCES

Alfonso, R. & Trigilio, J. (1997). Surfing the third wave: A dialogue between two third wave feminists. *Hypatia, 12*, 7-16.

B'nai B'rith Women. (1968). *Second Helpings Please.* Montreal, Canada: Mount Sinai Chapter #1091, B'nai B'rith Women.

Bailey, C. (1997). Making waves and drawing lines: The politics of defining the vicissitudes of feminism. *Hypatia, 12*, 17-28.

Bellafante, G. (1998, June 29). Feminism. It's all about me! *Time, 151,* 54-60.

Bondoc, A. (1995). Close, but no banana. In R. Walker (Ed.), *To Be Real* (pp. 167-184). New York: Anchor Books.

Chernik, A.F. (1995). The body politic. In B. Findlen (Ed.), *Listen Up: Voices From the Next Feminist Generation* (pp. 75-84). Seattle, Washington: Seal Press.

Damsky, L. (1998). Beauty Secrets. In O. Edut (Ed.), *Adiós Barbie: Young Women Write About Body Image and Identity* (pp. 133-143). Seattle, Washington: Seal Press.

Edut, O. (Ed.). (1998). *Adiós Barbie: Young Women Write About Body Image and Identity.* Seattle, Washington: Seal Press.

Findlen, B. (Ed.). (1995). *Listen Up: Voices From the Next Feminist Generation.* Seattle, Washington: Seal Press.

Lamm, N. (1995). It's a big fat revolution. In B. Findlen (Ed.), *Listen Up: Voices From the Next Feminist Generation* (pp. 85-94). Seattle, Washington: Seal Press.

Lamm, N. (1998). Fishnets, feather boas and fat. In O. Edut (Ed.), *Adiós Barbie: Young Women Write About Body Image and Identity.* (pp. 78-87). Seattle, Washington: Seal Press.

Morgan, D. (1995). Invisible women: Young women and feminism. In G. Griffin (Ed.), *Feminist Activism in the 1990's* (pp. 127-136). London: Taylor & Francis.

Nava, M. (1992). *Feminism, Youth, and Consumerism.* London: Sage Publications.

Navarro, M. (1998). Becoming La Mujer. In O. Edut (Ed.), *Adiós Barbie: Young Women Write About Body Image and Identity* (pp. 38-46). Seattle, Washington: Seal Press.

Orr, C.M. (1997). Charting the currents of the third wave. *Hypatia, 12,* 29-46.

Richards, A. (1998). Body image: Third wave feminism's issue? In O. Edut (Ed.), *Adiós Barbie: Young Women Write About Body Image and Identity* (pp. 196-201). Seattle, Washington: Seal Press.

Roiphe, K. (1993). *The Morning After: Sex, Fear, and Feminism on Campus.* Boston: Little, Brown, and Co.

Siegel, D. (1997). The legacy of the personal: Generating theory in feminism's third wave. *Hypatia, 12,* 46-75.

Walker, R. (Ed.). (1995). *To Be Real.* New York: Anchor Books.

Wolf, N. (1993). *Fire with Fire: The New Female Power and How it Will Change the 21st century.* New York: Random House.

Psychotherapy Partnership Approach with Adolescent Girls

Norine G. Johnson

SUMMARY. The Partnership Approach described in this article is designed to empower the adolescent girl in her own psychotherapy through a
process of shared decision-making. Through the integration of feminist
therapy tenets with current research on adolescent girls, the Partnership Approach focuses on valuing diversity and valuing strengths in today's adolescent girl clients, their families and their communities. *[Article copies available
for a fee from The Haworth Document Delivery Service: 1-800-342-9678. E-mail address:
<getinfo@haworthpressinc.com> Website: <http://www.HaworthPress.com> © 2001
by The Haworth Press, Inc. All rights reserved.]*

KEYWORDS. Adolescents, girls, feminist approaches

More girls want to come to therapy today than ever before. They still
bring the issues they always have: body image, relationships, conflict
with parents around issues of independence, school performance–but the
twist is different. The Psychotherapy Partnership Approach was designed
to meet the needs of today's adolescent girl by integrating feminist tenets
with current research on adolescent girls. The adolescent population in

Norine G. Johnson, PhD, is the 2001 President of the American Psychological Association. She is in private practice in Quincy, MA, where she specializes in adolescent
girls' and women's issues.
Address correspondence to: Norine G. Johnson, 110 W. Squantum Street, Quincy,
MA 02171.

[Haworth co-indexing entry note]: "Psychotherapy Partnership Approach with Adolescent Girls." Johnson, Norine G. Co-published simultaneously in *Women & Therapy* (The Haworth Press, Inc.) Vol. 23, No. 2,
2001, pp. 105-121; and: *The Next Generation: Third Wave Feminist Psychotherapy* (ed: Ellyn Kaschak) The
Haworth Press, Inc., 2001, pp. 105-121. Single or multiple copies of this article are available for a fee from
The Haworth Document Delivery Service [1-800-342-9678, 9:00 a.m. - 5:00 p.m. (EST). E-mail address:
getinfo@haworthpressinc.com].

the United States is growing rapidly and will continue to grow in this new millennium. These adolescents and their families need psychological services that are grounded in the current research and scholarship on gender, development, strength building, and race, ethnicity and culture. This article will provide a positive approach for psychotherapy with adolescent girls and is derivative of the scholarship challenging the accuracy of the stereotype of an inevitable, problematic adolescence (Offer, Ostrov, Howard, & Atkinson, 1988; Seligman, 1995; Worell & Danner, 1989). The partnership approach may be used in conjunction with other treatment approaches, e.g., cognitive/behavioral therapy, psychodynamically oriented therapy, and family therapy. Specific applications and case examples are given to illustrate the approach.

PSYCHOTHERAPY PARTNERSHIP APPROACH

The Partnership Approach is designed to empower the adolescent girl in her own psychotherapy. She becomes an equal partner in the process and participates in the decision-making process throughout the sessions. The partnership contract includes the adolescent girls' parents. The heart of the Partnership Approach is that most therapy decisions are shared decisions and that the process of making these decisions is explicit. Shared decisions include treatment and session goals, sequencing of the goals, aspects of confidentiality not covered by reporting mandates, appointment times, frequency and length of appointments, the participants at each session, and content and form of therapy.

The psychologist using the Partnership Approach is knowledgeable about the code of ethics of the American Psychological Association and always acts with a responsibility toward ethical behavior and the well being of her client. The Partnership Model does not give the treating psychologist permission to abdicate her responsibilities as a psychologist. The Partnership Model recognizes the power differential between the therapist and her client. The therapist is acknowledged as having informed knowledge and techniques. What the Partnership Model advocates is seeing that the client also has an informed knowledge base and that each–therapist and client–bring into the therapy special skills, knowledge, and strengths. Each partner, as in any good partnership, then strengthens the process by contributing her own areas of expertise.

PARTNERSHIP APPROACH VALUES

The Partnership Approach integrates tenets of feminist therapy (Wyche & Rice, 1997) with current research on adolescent girls. The research findings used in the partnership approach were part of the findings reported in *Beyond Appearance. A New Look at Adolescent Girls* (Johnson, Roberts, & Worell, 1999). This book is one of the products of the American Psychological Association's Presidential Task Force on Adolescent Girls which was initiated by Dr. Dorothy Cantor. The task force's mission was to explore why many adolescent girls are showing remarkable resiliency and strength during the stressful time of adolescence.

Consciousness-Raising Publications

The positive impact of books such as *Reviving Ophelia* (Pipher,1994) and the alarming, though flawed, research within the AAUW studies (1991, 1992) raised the American public's consciousness regarding the plight of adolescent girls. Dr. Pipher wrote compellingly about the impact of the media on the incidences of depression, eating disorders, suicide, and other mental health issues, with specific impact on teen girls. The AAUW 1992 study, showing a decline in self-esteem in girls as they approach adolescence, had a powerful impact on the research and discussion about adolescent girls. The AAUW research strongly suggested that schools were not providing appropriate environments for girls and hence were limiting their potential achievements.

However, this research was limited in important ways. It frequently generalized from the restricted lens of white skin privilege without acknowledging that limited perspective, and it focused on what was wrong, on problems rather than strengths. Also, the concept of adolescence as a time of stress continues to influence research and theory of adolescent development (Arnett, 1999).

Valuing Diversity and Valuing Strengths

The Partnership Approach focuses on valuing diversity and valuing strengths in today's adolescent girl clients, their families and their communities. Approximately one-third of the 18.5 million adolescent girls (ages 10-18), 6 million racial and ethnic minority girls, were living in the United States at the 1990 census (Oyhe & Daniel, 1999). Besides expertise on development, therapists must become knowledgeable about the ethnic and class cultures in our clients' communities. For teenagers, developing a consciousness and acceptance of the values and perspectives of their culture aids their development of a personal identity.

By focusing on strengths and encouraging the client's active participation, the Partnership Approach represents a primary feminist value. (Johnson, 1995; Wyche & Rice, 1997). The social construction of gender within the framework of strengths facilitates adolescent girls viewing their world within context, rather than as personal failures. The therapist who focuses on strengths will use the principles of feminist and womanist psychology to help girls understand the effect of society's racism, sexism, classism. The therapist will focus on helping the girl both be independent and stay connected, to enact and endure, to use her strengths and agency in the development of her creativity, athletic abilities, relationships, career opportunities, and cognitive abilities.

Looking at strengths rather than deficits, opportunities rather than risks, assets rather than liabilities is slowly becoming an increasing presence in the psychotherapy, education, and parenting literature. Looking at strengths does not deny the difficulty of the passage of adolescence, but rather asserts that strength-based interventions approach the stresses by building competencies, enhancing connections, and empowering the adolescent (Bertolino, 1999; Dryfoos, 1998).

APPLICATIONS OF THE PARTNERSHIP APPROACH TO PSYCHOTHERAPY

Specific therapeutic applications of the Partnership Approach will be the focus of the next section. These include methods for establishing a therapeutic contract regarding the goals, content, and form of therapy that empowers the adolescent girl, shared decision-making on issues such as confidentiality and session participants, and valuing diversity and building strengths.

Strengths Inventory

Because most standard diagnostic forms and tools lack breadth in assessing a girl's strengths, it is recommended that therapists utilizing the partnership approach supplement their standard intake forms with a strengths assessment. This author has found the following Strengths Inventory helpful. (See Table 1.)

TABLE 1. Assessment of Strengths Inventory*
Norine G. Johnson, PhD

1. LIST FIVE (5) AREAS OF STRENGTH YOU SEE IN YOURSELF.
2. LIST FIVE (5) AREAS OF STRENGTH THAT OTHERS SAID ABOUT YOU WHEN YOU WERE YOUNGER.
3. LIST FIVE (5) THINGS YOU DO THAT GIVE YOU SATISFACTION.
4. LIST FIVE (5) THINGS YOU DO THAT SOOTHE YOU WHEN ANXIOUS, ANGRY, OR SAD.
5. LIST FIVE (5) PEOPLE YOU THINK SHOWED STRENGTH.
6. LIST FIVE (5) THINGS YOU LIKE ABOUT YOUR APPEARANCE AND YOUR BODY.
7. LIST FIVE (5) POSITIVE THINGS YOUR BEST FRIEND WOULD SAY ABOUT YOU.

* Copyright 1998.

After the initial session the girl client is asked to take the form home and return it at the following appointment. Depending upon the age of the client, after each question the form includes 3 to 5 lines for the client's answers. It is not usual for teen girls entering therapy to leave blanks on the inventory form. Re-administering the inventory after the fifth, tenth and final sessions may be used as one outcome measure.

Initial Session with Girl

Defining the Partnership Approach begins early with an adolescent girl. During the introductory session as part of the initial decision about working together, the Partnership Approach is described. "The work we do together is like a partnership. Therapy is not something that is done to you. I see therapy as us working together." Some girls, more likely an early teen, 10-13, object to the word "therapy" and with these girls we change the description of what we do together to "talks." In fact, this is an example of an early working of the partnership. The therapist is willing to give up the word "therapy" and replace it with another word upon which both agree.

Also, at the beginning of therapy, the teen and her family are told that she may invite anyone to the session she wishes, that this is her time. The limits of the invitation are explained, including that if the guest is someone under the legal age of consent there must be signed parental consent, that the therapist can not be the guest's therapist, and that the limits of confidentiality apply also to the guest. The following case example is a brief description of the range of flexibility of session participants that may be used by a girl client:

> *Case example.* Sue was referred for depression as a reaction to a life-threatening disease. She was an exceptionally bright girl from an intact, loving family. She had a great personality and before her depression, a strong sense of self. During the course of our two year therapy, she brought to therapy: her mother, her mother and father, her younger sister, and her boyfriend. She also brought two of her boyfriend's friends. They came to one session because one of the friends had confided that he was sexually abused by his uncle and they wanted to support him.

In this approach, defining the work as a partnership is a tangible step in empowering the adolescent girl and making concrete the responsibility she has. She is asked from the beginning to let the therapist know if the therapeutic approach is working for her. She is told there is no one way to do therapy or "talk," that what is important is for her and the therapist to find what works best. She is told that some research about how girls build strengths, feel better about themselves, and have more connected relationships will be discussed.

Treatment and Session Goals

The general treatment goals are a shared decision made by the parents, the adolescent girl and the therapist. However, prioritizing of the goals changes over time and is the responsibility of the participants at each session. Maintaining a working relationship with adolescents is facilitated when the girls participate actively in setting the session goals. Some teen girls, however, will carry the "nice girl" role into therapy and may defer to their parents or the therapist regarding specific goals. For these girls the empowerment of them, session by session, to decide treatment goals reinforces that this is a partnership and that they are key players. For many therapists, this may not be different from what they do daily. However, what is different is that this procedure is explained explicitly at the beginning of therapy to both the parents and the teen client.

> *Case example.* Two years ago a fifteen-year-old girl was referred for therapy by her school counselor. The counselor described the

girl by using a plethora of diagnoses: multi-drug and alcohol use, depression, school failure, conduct disorder, and thought disorder. She was unsuccessful in school and was placed in an alternative class. She had no friends. Her mother also had experienced trauma. Then I met Lisa. She was wonderful. Straightforward. Let me know what she wanted to talk about and what she didn't. She did not want to talk about family. She wanted to talk about the friends she had before she moved to Boston and how she missed them. And she wanted to talk about what "level" she was on and how she could get to the next "level." So that's what we talked about until she was ready to talk about the almost unbearable trauma in her life. In our therapeutic contract, I respected Lisa's ability and right to set the agenda and to determine the content of each session and the pace at which she approached painful material.

Participants in Sessions

The Partnership Approach takes as a high priority fostering a more positive relationship between the adolescent girl and her parents. Therefore, not including the mother and father in the therapy with an adolescent girl should be the exception, not the rule. In the Partnership Approach, the therapist will work collaboratively with the entire family, making decisions as to what will be the most effective way to foster the relationships and, if there has been a rift, to do reparative work. The younger adolescent girl is frequently more open to this work. Girls in early and middle adolescence frequently yearn to reconnect with their mothers emotionally, if the re-connection doesn't mean giving up hard-fought battles for independence.

Mothers

The quality of a girl's interaction with her mother is an important predictor of a girl's self-esteem and her general health (Resnick et al., 1997). Therefore, to leave the mother out of the therapy is counter-indicated. When there is already a positive relationship between the girl and her parents, and the girl wants to deal with other issues such as peer relationships and her own emerging self, it may be appropriate to see the girl for individual psychotherapy. However, the therapist using the partnership approach will continue to monitor the family relationships and work out a contract with the girl by which her parents may stay appropriately informed about the general course of therapy. The strong findings about the importance of a teen girl's relationships with both her mother and father challenge a therapeutic model that only includes individual psychotherapy. The old standard that therapeutic work with teenagers cannot include parents is simply not true for therapists with family therapy skills. In fact, the Partnership Model avows that therapy with a teen must include therapeutic involvement of the parents in order to achieve the therapeutic goals. The issue is not whether to include the parents, but how. In order to build positive relationships among all members of an adolescent girl's family, it is imperative that the parents, both mother and father, agree to be full participants in the sessions. The various options are obviously individual and/or family therapy or sharing the work with another therapist. There is no set combination for all girls. The treatment modality needs to be flexible to represent the changing needs of the teen girl and her family. For example, treatment might start with individual work with the girl, then dyad work with the mother and daughter, then dyad work with the father and daughter, and finally family work with all three or even the entire family including siblings.

Case example. Lucy's parents were concerned with her isolation from the family, her rudeness, her grades, her behavior in school, and her poor relationships with her siblings. She did not want to be in therapy. She thought it was "dumb." She wanted her parents to "leave me alone." The one key piece she gave me, from her curled position inside the frame of my office chair, was that her parents were impossibly protective.

Under the partnership framework, Lucy and I and her parents agreed on a format in which Lucy and I would meet for the first half of the session and then her mother would join us. Lucy would not let her father join the sessions for three months. During this time Lucy and her mother focused on how early traumatic deaths in the family had affected their relationship. Mother worked very hard on her anxiety and over-protectiveness. They developed contractual agreements on curfew, attendance at meals, and homework. As Lucy began sharing her learning experiences and feelings about how she learned, a learning disorder was suggested and later confirmed with a neuropsychological evaluation. At first it was hard for the parents to give Lucy control of certain decisions but as they did they found she participated more at home.

Fathers

A girl's relationship with her father contributes significantly to the development of her feelings about herself as a woman and her future leadership skills (Cantor & Bernay, 1992; Resnick et al., 1997). Fathers have a critical role in the life of today's adolescent girls. The new psychology of men explores how society's expectations for men contribute to men's difficulties with their emotional lives and with their relationships (Betcher & Pollack, 1993; Brooks, 1998; Levant, 1992). A therapist using the Partnership Approach will be aware of the gender issues of men as well as women.

The supportive connected father helps his daughter develop a positive attitude toward herself and her abilities. Using the Partnership Approach the therapist sees the entire family as "the client" and she will assess the father's ability to form a positive relationship with his daughter that includes communicating about feelings, tolerance for his daughter's increasing independence, and comfort with her sexuality. The therapist is aware when a father is unable to be in touch with his own feelings, to modulate his anxiety about his daughter's sexuality, or when a father is angry and sees his daughter's increasing independence as disrespect. For some girl clients, there is a direct connection between their depression and the experience of a poor relationship with their fathers.

The following is excerpted from the initial interview with an adolescent girl presenting with symptoms of depression.

> *Case example.* "I'm never very, very happy. I feel happy sometimes, then feel lonely and upset. It's [the depression] been around awhile. I think I've always had it. I'm annoyed with my family. I never want to be around them. My friends understand me. My mom says, 'How's school?' and I don't want to talk about it. Same feeling with Dad. No, it's usually my Dad. I have my friends and my family and I don't want to mix them. My Dad doesn't trust me. There were a few incidents with his finding beer cans. He said I had to tell him who drank them. He made me rat on my friend. If I didn't, I'd be grounded for the summer. I had to choose between him and my friends. I have two best friends. Molly. I talk to her a lot. And David. He's a senior and he's going to college. I'm a

sophomore. My Dad says you shouldn't be close to your friends who are going away."

Terence Real (1997) writes about the "secret legacy of men's depression" and focuses on the concept of lovingly holding men accountable, a perspective on men as "wounded wounders." In this example, the father denied and projected his anxiety about the potential loss of his daughter. Rather than owning his own feelings, he told his daughter not to be close to her friends because she would lose them when they go to college. He gave her a message that felt like, "Choose me, not your friends." But he couldn't see his fear of being alone, of her growing up, or her leaving him. He wounded her under the guise of protecting her.

In working with this family it was important for the therapist to make a partnership contract with the father, mother and the teen girl. Understanding the gender issues of a woman treating a male client will help the therapist working with a teen's father (Johnson, in press). The father was open to reading a book about men's psychology and to discussing how his father treated his sisters. Both he and the mother were informed about research on the importance of helping a girl become independent, as a way to protect her.

The Breakfast Club has been a successful approach for several fathers to use in establishing or re-establishing a connection to their teen daughter. Saturday mornings, sometime between 10 and 12, several fathers and their teen daughters have breakfast at a local coffee shop. It is time-limited and seems to fit with the hectic schedules of today's families. The Partnership Approach encourages special time for the teen girl and each parent. With the exception of involvement in the girls' sporting activities, girls and their mothers seem to find more activities in common than teen girls and their fathers. Therefore, a time once a month or bi-monthly that becomes a looked forward to routine can provide a time for dad and daughter just to be together and to learn to talk together.

FORM AND CONTENT OF PARTNERSHIP APPROACH PSYCHOTHERAPY

The content of sessions with adolescent girls is informed by the current scholarship and research. Universal issues are ethnicity and racism, body image and gender, developing competencies, other "mothers" and "fathers," giving voice, and developing independence.

Ethnic Identity and Racism

Using the Partnership Approach a therapist will devise applications that value the cultural, social, political, economic and historical context of her client and the client's family. These applications will include strengths represented in that culture as girls from different ethnicities, races, and classes use different standards to judge themselves and have different strengths (Erkut et al., 1996). For example, in working with African-American, Asian-American, and Mexican-American teens, the therapist who assists the girl in searching for or obtaining her ethnic identity will help her attain increased self-esteem (Phinney, 1990; Phinney & Rosenthal, 1992).

Under the Partnership Model the topic of racism may be introduced by either the girl or the therapist but the therapist recognizes the importance of having the conversation. Sometimes such a conversation may start with an incident that appears minor. But how the therapist handles this will set the tone for the adolescent girl to share more of her experiences of a racist society. Here is how one Korean-American client began what turned into several sessions of her increasing disclosure of the racism she experienced in her suburban community. The conversation started by asking her about racism in her school and community. She responded with anger about being seen in a racially stereotyped way that has nothing to do with her or her abilities.

> *Case example.* "It really makes me mad. I don't experience it with my friends. But it happens all the time with people who don't know me. They say things to me like 'You're just a whiz in math.' I hate math and I'm not very good at it."

Body Image and Gender

Using the Partnership Approach a feminist therapist assesses the body image of her clients from the perspective of knowing the pressures society places on girls and that processes of socio-cultural gendering will influence the formation of self-esteem, self-competency, and perceptions of the physical, sexual, and social self (Balentine et al., 1991; Macpherson & Fine, 1995; Yoder, 1999). It is important to know and hear how the girl sees herself, the pressures she feels, what she can acknowledge as positive aspects of her appearance. Also important are the attitudes of her parents regarding body type and food.

Using the Partnership Approach means helping a girl see the positive aspects of her appearance. The therapist will educate the girl and her family on the role of gender in today's society and how the societal images and pressures have a negative impact on girls' self image. The following is a case example of a therapist using the Partnership Approach who joined with a client on the cusp of physical change who did not like the changes. The girl liked her previously lean, hard body and was disappointed with the failure of that promised glory of womanhood.

> *Case example.* I saw Alex when she was 11 years old. Her mother is a former anorectic who does not want her daughter to suffer as she did. The mother is striking at 5'8"with long blonde hair, articulate, self-assured, and thin, very thin. Her child is charming, bright, intelligent, creative, warm, spontaneous, and chunky, very chunky. In an early session Alex described herself. "My body is changing and I don't like it. They told me I would be beautiful. I like my body the way it was–hard." Over this year of therapy Alex's body hasn't changed. What has changed is that she now has friends and perhaps a different way of looking at herself. Recently she said, "I like the way I look. My dad and I had a talk. He said, I'm like he was as a teen and that he outgrew it and I would too."

Starting in early adolescence, the influence of gender intensifies. Conceptions about gender roles and gender identity and how they measure up as developing women move into new focus during adolescence. Gender is the earliest marker of "differences" in the development of girls. Understanding the impact of gender requires the therapist using the Partnership Approach to analyze the power relationships in her girl client's life.

Developing Competencies

Although girls achieve at a level equal to or better than boys in most areas, by early adolescence they may begin to doubt their abilities, and achievement declines (AAUW, 1991). This decline occurs especially in math and science, but for some girls it cuts across areas. At all ages, girls' expectancies for success tend to be lower than their abilities and they tend to underestimate their competency in many areas. In contrast, more girls are entering sports and asserting their right to compete in any sphere of life.

The therapist using the Partnership Model will survey the teen girl's areas of competency and help her client increase her appreciation of her skills and competencies. Frequently this requires a structured program whereby the girl gradually tries different activities and areas of study until she finds the "right fit." In using the Partnership Approach it is crucial for the therapist not just to explore the teen's emotional distress and relationship difficulties. The Partnership Approach focuses on helping the girl re-visualize herself through her strengths and her competencies. The therapist may serve briefly as a coach during this time.

The Partnership Model means consulting to school systems when appropriate for a teen client. In order to be an effective consultant the therapist better serves her client by knowing the research about teaching methods and institutions of learning for girls. For example, if a teen girl expresses an interest in developing competencies in either science or the Internet, her therapist will want to have the parents investigate the accessibility of her school's advanced science courses for girls (Farmer, 1985). In the counseling of parents of girls who show an interest and talent in science, the Partnership Approach helps the parents support their girls' aspirations and teaches the parents how to advocate within the school for girl-friendly teaching. Research findings that show gender bias in Computer Science (AAUW, 2000) can alert parents to the advocacy they need to do in their communities.

Other "Mothers" and "Fathers"

Recent research confirms what we already knew but perhaps under-appreciated: the impact of adults in the lives of adolescent girls, not only mothers and fathers, but "other mothers" such as extended family members, family friends, and others. Using the Partnership Approach the feminist therapist will inquire about the adults her girl client has available for advice, support, and guidance as she negotiates her place in the wider culture. Some of the questions the therapist will want to pose to her teen client are, Whom does she trust? Is there an adult relative, teacher, mother of a friend, priest, etc., available to her? Was she betrayed by adults who turned away? Has she lost a significant woman, perhaps her grandmother? The therapist needs to ask herself, Is it appropriate for me to temporarily be an "other mother"?

The availability of appropriate spiritual role models is related to a healthy self-concept in adolescent girls. The Partnership Approach assesses the availability of spiritual role models and mentors for the teen girl. Girls who may not attend a religious institution regularly frequently have their own spirituality. The therapist needs to join with the teen girl who is exploring her spirituality. This may mean reading books or other material important to the girl. The Partnership Approach encourages the therapist to understand the religious models of her teen clients by knowing the community's religious institutions and leaders.

Giving Voice

As Mary Pipher (1994) identified, the pressures and dangers are more intense today for adolescent girls. These girls know that to thrive today they must be strong and to be strong they must be prepared to be active decision-makers and participants. Sometimes their parents do not know how to prepare their daughters for the changes in society. Their parents are fear-bound and want their daughters to be "good girls" in a day when being a good girl isn't enough. It doesn't even keep you safe anymore.

A principle of the Partnership Approach is the empowerment of women and girls. The ability to be outspoken in relationships promotes strength and resiliency in girls. Girls who are outspoken in relationships have been found to be strong and resilient (Taylor et al., 1995; Way, 1995). Way's research reaffirms the importance of assessing our girl clients' "voice" and teaching assertion skills to these girls. By adolescence relationships with friends and peers take central stage and become a fundamental source of influence and support (Brown & Gilligan, 1992). Therapists using the Partnership Approach will actively structure sessions and devise exercises to help girls find and keep their voice in all relationships.

The Partnership Approach involves the girl and her family in the promotion of social change. Helping girls and their parents develop the skills to prevent sexual harassment or deal with it when it occurs are one example of what a therapist and family might contract to do. Working in partnership with adolescent girls to promote social change will involve working in the girls' communities and their schools. Teacher training and parent groups provide opportunities for sharing the research and approaches available to promote healthy and safe school environments for girls and boys.

The Supreme Court ruled that school districts can be liable for damages for failing to stop a student from subjecting another to severe, pervasive, and objectively offensive sexual harassment behavior. For feminist therapists this was another acknowledgment of the stresses and hazards that adolescent girls face in environments that should be safe for them. Sharing significant statistics with school, parent and/or teacher groups can provide a wake-up call. A good beginning is to encourage parents to ask what their schools' policies on sexual harassment are.

Developing Independence

Problem-solving skills that demonstrate independence and family support for independence help lead a girl through barriers during her adolescence. Girls need problem-solving skills that foster independence in many arenas of their lives. Sexuality and sexual harassment are major areas of potential conflict and trauma for teen girls. A therapist using the Partnership Approach will help her girl client develop her own attitudes about sexuality and skills for handling harassment. In empowering parents and their teen girls to work together to achieve appropriate independence, it can be helpful to share relevant statistics. Providing data and research findings treats the clients like a partner and facilitates the transition into a discussion about how to immunize their daughter to the risks in today's world.

By focusing parents on the girl's need for independent skills by the time she is graduated from high school and leaves home for either work or college, they come to understand the importance of helping her develop coping skills for independent living. It is the girl's responsibility to learn the problem-solving strategies to advance her independence while keeping safe.

CONCLUSION

The Partnership Approach described in this article is designed to empower the adolescent girl in her own psychotherapy through a process of shared decision-making. Through the integration of feminist therapy tenets with current research on adolescent girls the Partnership Approach focuses on valuing diversity and valuing strengths in today's adolescent girl clients, their families, and their communities.

REFERENCES

American Association of University Women. (1991). *Shortchanging girls, shortchanging America.* Washington, DC: American Association of University Women Educational Foundation.
American Association of University Women. (1992). *How schools shortchange girls: Study of major findings on girls and education.* Washington, DC: American Association of University Women Educational Foundation.

American Association of University Women. (2000) Tech-savvy: Educating girls in the new computer age. Washington, DC: American Association of University Women Foundation Research.

Arnett, J. (1999). Adolescent storm and stress, reconsidered. *American Psychologist, 54*, 317-326.

Balentine, M., Stitt, K., Bonner, J., & Clark, L. (1991). Self-reported eating disorders of black, low-income adolescents: Behavior, body weight perceptions, and methods of dieting. *Journal of School Health, 61*, 392-396.

Bertolino, B. (1999). *Therapy with troubled teenagers: Rewriting young lives in progress.* NY: John Wiley & Sons.

Betcher, W. & Pollack, W. (1993). *In a time of fallen heroes: The re-creation of masculinity.* New York: Macmillian Publishing Company.

Brooks, G. (1998). *A new psychotherapy for traditional men.* San Francisco: Jossey-Bass Publishers.

Brown, L.M. & Gilligan, C. (1992). *Meeting at the crossroads: Women's psychology and girls' development.* Cambridge, MA: Harvard University Press.

Cantor, D.W. & Bernay, T. (1992). "Women in Power: The Secrets of Leadership." Boston: HoughtonMifflin.

Dryfoos, J. (1998). *Making it through adolescence in a risky society: What parents, schools, and communities can do.* New York: Oxford University Press.

Erkut, S., Fields, J., Sing, R., & Marx, F. (1996). Diversity in girls' experiences: Feeling good about who you are. In B.R. Leadbeater & N. Way (Eds.), *Urban Girls: Resisting stereotypes, creating identities.* (pp 53-64). New York: NYU Press.

Farmer, F. (1985). A model of career and achievement motivation for women and men. *Journal of Counseling Psychology, 32*, 363-390.

Johnson, N.G. (1995, August). Feminist frames of women's strength: Visions for the future. Presidential Address to the Division of the Psychology of Women, presented at the Annual Convention of the American Psychological Association's, New York, NY.

Johnson, N.G. (In press). Women helping men: Strengths of and barriers to women therapists working with men clients. In G. Brooks & G. Good, *The handbook of counseling and psychotherapy approaches for men.* San Francisco: Jossey-Bass.

Johnson, N.G., Roberts, M.C., & Worell, J. (Eds.) 1999. *Beyond appearance: A new look at adolescent girls.* Washington, DC: American Psychological Association.

Levant, R. (1992). Toward the reconstruction of masculinity. *Journal of Family Psychology, 5* (3&4), 379-402.

Macpherson, P. & Fine, M. (1995). Hungry for an us: Adolescent girls and women negotiating territories of race, gender, and class difference. *Feminism and Psychology, 5*, 181-200.

Offer, D., Ostrov, E., Howard, K.I., & Atkinson, R. (1988). *The teenager: Adolescents' self image in ten countries.* (pp. 115-129). New York: Plenum Medical Book Company.

Ohye, B. & Daniel, J. (1999). The "other" adolescent girls: Who are they? In N.G. Johnson, M.C. Roberts & J. Worell (Eds.), *Beyond appearance: A new look at adolescent girls.* Washington, DC: American Psychological Association.

Phinney, J.S. (1990). Ethnic identity in adolescents and adults: Review of research. *Psychological Bulletin, 108*, 449-514.

Phinney, J.S. & Rosenthal, D.A. (1992). Ethnic identity in adolescence: Process, context, and outcome. In G. R. Adams, T.P. Gullotta, & R. Montemayor (Eds.) *Adolescent identity formation* (pp. 145-172). Newbury Park, CA: Sage.

Pipher, M. (1994). *Reviving Ophelia: Saving the selves of adolescent girls.* New York: Ballantine Books.

Real, T. (1997). *I don't want to talk about it: Overcoming the secret legacy of male depression.* New York: Scribner.

Resnick, M.D., Bearman, P.S., Blum, R.W., Bauman, K.E., Harris, K.M., Jones, J., Tabor, J., Beuhring, T., Sieving, R.E., Shew, M., Ireland, M., Bearinger, L.H., & Udry, J.R. (1997). Protecting adolescents from harm: Findings from the National Longitudinal Study on Adolescent Health. *Journal of the American Medical Association, 278,* 823-832.

Seligman, M. E. (1995). *The optimistic child.* New York: Houghton Mifflin Company.

Striegel-Moore, R. & Cachelin, F. (1999). Body image concerns and disordered eating in adolescent girls: Risk and protective factors. In N.G. Johnson, M.C. Roberts & J. Worell (Eds.), *Beyond appearance: A new look at adolescent girls.* Washington, DC: American Psychological Association.

Taylor, J., Gilligan, C., & Sullivan, A. (1995). *Between voice and silence: Women and girls, race and relationship.* Cambridge, MA: Harvard University Press.

Way, N. (1995). "Can't you see the courage, the strength that I have?" : Listening to urban adolescent girls speak about their relationship. *Psychology of Women Quarterly, 19,* 107-128.

Worell, J. & Danner, F. (1989). Adolescents in contemporary context. In J.Worell and F. Danner (Eds.), *The adolescent as decision-maker* (pp. 3-12). San Diego, CA: Academic Press.

Worell, J. & Remer, P. (1992). *Feminist perspectives in therapy: An empowerment model for women.* New York: Wiley and Sons, Inc.

Worell, J. & Johnson, N.G. (Eds.). 1997. *Shaping the future of feminist psychology: Research, education, and practice.* Washington, DC: American Psychological Association.

Wyche, K. & Rice, J. (1997). Feminist therapy: From dialogue to tenets. In J. Worell and N. Johnson (Eds.). *Shaping the future of feminist psychology: Education, research, and practice* (57-71). Washington, DC: American Psychological Association.

Yoder, J. (1999). *Women and gender: Transforming psychology.* Upper Saddle River, NJ: Prentice Hall.

Index

For Product Safety Concerns and Information please contact our EU
representative GPSR@taylorandfrancis.com Taylor & Francis Verlag GmbH,
Kaufingerstraße 24, 80331 München, Germany

Printed and bound by CPI Group (UK) Ltd, Croydon, CR0 4YY
01/05/2025
01858509-0002